The International Library of Sociology

SOCIAL SERVICE AND MENTAL HEALTH

Founded by KARL MANNHEIM

The International Library of Sociology

THE SOCIOLOGY OF MENTAL HEALTH

In 7 Volumes

I	The Desegregation of the Mentally Ill	*Hoenig et al*
II	Lunacy, Law, and Conscience	*Jones*
III	Mental Health and Social Policy 1845 - 1959	*Jones*
IV	Mental Hospitals at Work	*Jones et al*
V	Psychiatric Social Work in Great Britain (1939 - 1962)	*Timms*
VI	Put Away	*Morris*
VII	Social Service and Mental Health	*Ashdown et al*

SOCIAL SERVICE AND MENTAL HEALTH

An Essay on Psychiatric Social Workers

by
MARGARET ASHDOWN
and
S. CLEMENT BROWN

ROUTLEDGE
Taylor & Francis Group

First published in 1953 by
Routledge and Kegan Paul Ltd

Reprinted 1996, 2000 by
Routledge
11 New Fetter Lane, London EC4P 4EE

Routledge is an imprint of the Taylor & Francis Group

Printed and bound in Great Britain

British Library Cataloguing in Publication Data
A CIP catalogue record for this book
is available from the British Library

Social Service and Mental Health
ISBN 0-415-17808-8
The Sociology of Mental Health: 7 Volumes
ISBN 0-415-17835-5
The International Library of Sociology: 274 Volumes
ISBN 0-415-17838-X

PREFACE

THIS book is about individuals who choose and are chosen for psychiatric social work, the use that they make of training and the shaping of their careers when they enter employment.

In so far as it is concerned with our direct experience the book refers exclusively to one course of training during a limited period of time. The fact that the special study round which it is written was confined to women cannot be without influence on the book as a whole. We regard men as important to the profession and consider that training of this kind has greater value when men and women are trained together. We could however only have done justice to the special circumstances affecting men if our study had been on a far larger scale. They were therefore regretfully omitted.

We hope that readers will not be confused by traces of the passing of time. This applies to the period at which individual subjects of the special study undertook their training and also to the survey of their subsequent employment. More than five years have passed since the book was planned. Within this period many changes have been taking place in the careers in which we have been interested, in the profession itself and in the mental health and other services. But the broader themes which have isolated themselves as the book progressed seem to us to be largely independent of this influence.

The advantages and disadvantages of the close personal concern which we ourselves had in the training we have described will be obvious, as will those attendant upon any form of collaboration in writing.

In connexion with the special study described in the book we wish to thank the London School of Economics and its Director for access to records, and all who, with such generous readiness, took part in the study as 'subjects' or 'referees'. We would also acknowledge the help of many professional colleagues, both in academic and practical work, with whom we have discussed what we were doing from time to time. Our debt to Eileen Younghusband is of a special kind, since we have not only had the great advantage of drawing upon her valuable reports undertaken for the Carnegie Trust[1] but of receiving her personal advice and encouragement. We should like also to mention with special appreciation the encouragement both in our work and in our writing of Professor Aubrey Lewis and Professor T. H. Marshall. We are grateful for the general support of the Association of Psychiatric Social Workers in our endeavour, for the outcome of which they have of course no responsibility. We shall feel that some small return has been made if the book provides the Association with topics for lively controversy. All former students of the London Mental Health Course whom we have taught and through and with whom we have learned (whether or not they are members of the Association) have unwittingly put us in their debt. It is they indeed who are the 'true begetters' of this book.

We are deeply indebted to N. Newbigin and to the anonymous contributor of another of the case studies in Chapter III, who have added much to the value of this book.

We would express our thanks to all who have granted us permission to quote from published material. For our general ideas we have obviously drawn upon a much wider range of sources than our few references indicate.

[1] Younghusband, Eileen L.: *Report on the Employment and Training of Social Workers* and *Social Work in Britain* (Supplementary Report), Carnegie United Kingdom Trust, 1947 and 1951.

CONTENTS

CHAPTER I

INTRODUCTION

WITHIN the present century the work people do, the suitability of different people for different types of work and the equipment needed to undertake them have all been subjected to a new kind of scrutiny. Work has been lifted out of its natural surroundings in the whole process of living and broken up into problems to be analysed. This has come about to a great extent for sternly practical reasons, not least those rooted in two world wars.[1] But if, when the conception of work is examined, the community's demand for the contribution of the individual takes first place, there is always present another consideration—the personal satisfaction which work affords to the individual, as an expression of his abilities and an assurance to himself of being needed by his fellows. This conception is certainly implicit in vocational guidance, which is concerned with serenity as a personal matter, as well as with the fact that if someone is, and feels himself to be, suited to the work he is doing, he is likely to make his best contribution to society. The converging of these two approaches is well illustrated by the investigation of the Industrial Health Research Board of the Medical Research Council reported in 1947 under the title of *The Incidence of Neurosis Among Factory Workers.*[2]

There are questions common to the whole range of work, from manual work, where the chief emphasis falls upon the breaking up of processes so that they may be carried out in the most economical way, to the professions, where emphasis might be said to fall

[1] The effect of the last war in advancing knowledge in the spheres of selection of individuals for jobs, methods of training and job analysis is described in a report, Privy Council Office: *The Work of Psychologists and Psychiatrists in the Services*, H.M. Stationery Office, 1947. This matter is further discussed in Chapter IV, p. 55.

[2] Fraser, Russell (*et al.*): Medical Research Council, Industrial Health Research Board, Report No. 90, *The Incidence of Neurosis Among Factory Workers*, H.M. Stationery Office, 1947.

almost evenly upon selection, training and practice. Valuable investigations have been undertaken in all three spheres, but, as far as we are aware, there exist few studies in which selection, training and practice are considered as an indivisible sequence,[1] in terms of the person who chooses a particular form of work.

The writers[2] of this book belong to a group of professions where the lack of such studies is especially unfortunate. These are the professions where practitioners, in direct contact with individual human beings, undertake to meet particular needs. We take this group to include, for example, the medical practitioner, the solicitor, the fully qualified social worker, but not the accountant or the engineer. In these professions the welfare of two sets of human beings is in the most intimate sense at stake, of those who enter and qualify and those whose needs they are prepared to serve. Those who take upon themselves to select candidates and to launch them into these professions with suitable equipment are making a large claim. To say to those who have chosen a certain form of service 'you may' or 'you may not' train for it is to assume a serious responsibility. There may be gains as well as losses in allowing individuals to try and fail in their chosen employment, though the losses are more evident than the gains. Those who are called upon to undertake such responsibilities need the support of any obtainable knowledge.

If one were looking for an ideal field of study one would be unlikely to turn to one of the older professions, with their tangled history and complicated structure. One would look rather for a profession not too long established or too large, and simple in structure. It would be an advantage if its members could be counted upon to help in the study and had already given thought to some of the questions which it was proposed to explore. We believe that the profession to which we belong to a great extent

[1] A long term pilot study, initiated in 1947 by the New York School of Social Work to establish criteria for selecting candidates for social work, is planned to follow students into employment (referred to in S. Berengarten's 'A Pioneer Workshop in Student Selection', Bulletin of New York School of Social Work, July 1951).

[2] In a book as dependent as this on personal experience, it has seemed most convenient and most honest to write in the first person. The plural 'we' simply represents our collaboration; we hope it has no royal or editorial flavour. Because we are part of what we write of, 'we' sometimes comes to mean the profession of psychiatric social workers. Occasionally we have fallen into the conventional usage of associating reader and writer under the formal 'we', where these are assumed to be in accord.

fulfils these conditions.[1] Psychiatric social work was established in this country a little over twenty years ago. In January 1951 the membership of its professional association was just over 450 and, although its increasing numbers begin to make it a more impersonal body, it still has something of its earlier intimacy. Moreover, the nature of the work and the pressure of external events have served to keep alive in its members an interest in recruitment, selection and training in relation to the wide variety of work which those who qualify are called upon to undertake. Here, it would seem, is a field for a study which, on however modest a scale, might yield results with some bearing upon other professions faced with the same essentially human problems.

In 1947 both of us, after some fifteen years on the staff of the Mental Health Course of the London School of Economics, one of the three professional training courses for psychiatric social work, had ceased to be associated with the Course, and were moreover no longer directly employed in this work. During these fifteen years one of us, as tutor, had been stationed at the centre of the training, not only representing its academic aspect but responsible for general planning and for keeping a balance between its various elements. The other had worked chiefly on the circumference, in a clinical setting, with responsibility for the supervision of students' practical training in work with adult patients. Our posts had thus been complementary, allowing us to view our common field from different standpoints. Of the three phases which we proposed to consider—selection, training and practice—it was in the second that our own work had chiefly lain, although both of us had also been concerned in selection. With regard to practice, we had between us kept some contact with many of those who had passed through the London Mental Health Course up to 1947, and in one way or another had learned a good deal about the work that was being done by former students in this country and overseas.

Without further effort we thus had a considerable store upon which to draw. We might have written, as it is sometimes best to do in the case of a special experience, exclusively out of the knowledge and impressions which had come to us unsought. But what individual experience provides is in a sense fortuitous, and certainly limited. We were aware that aspects of the problems which former students had been facing in the field had necessarily eluded us.

[1] In a later chapter we discuss some of the reasons for including psychiatric social work among the professions.

Moreover, our earlier position on the training staff, while giving us access to useful sources of information, was likely to have restricted our view in certain directions. Our experience of training, the area where our knowledge was most comprehensive, was inevitably one-sided, and our collaboration only reduced to a very limited degree the danger that what we encountered was not characteristic and that our interpretation was subject to bias.

When therefore we found ourselves free from any official connexion with the London Mental Health Course, it occurred to us that we might be able to enlarge and adjust our own range of ideas about all three phases of psychiatric social work by tapping the experience and views of former students. Now perhaps, when we could be regarded as disinterested persons, they would feel able to talk to us with greater freedom about the professional problems on which we were all seeking enlightenment. We felt confident that psychiatric social workers as a whole would be interested in such a proposal and would wish to help. We planned to combine our own experiences with a study of some of the students who had passed through the London Mental Health Course, in which we should trace their careers from selection, through training, out into employment. The comparatively small number of subjects whom we finally decided to include ruled out the possibility of dealing with the material from a quantitative standpoint. This was of less importance in that the questions which had chiefly stirred our interest were not to be answered in statistical terms.

As our sample we decided to take students who trained during the four sessions lying between 1935 and 1939. In this way we avoided the earliest years, when conditions of selection and training had not settled into the shape which became characteristic of the Course, and also the war years, when conditions of selection, training and practice were all unusual. We simplified our study by excluding overseas students and also men.[1] We then made a mechanical adjustment so that the sample might be more representative of the Course as a whole in such matters as age on entry and qualification before admission. The adjusted sample numbered sixty-four. To this we added two groups drawn from all but the earliest years of the Course down to the time when our study began; these consisted of students, not already included in the

[1] Of the eight men students trained within the sample years, three are employed as psychiatric social workers. Several returned to the posts of Borstal housemasters from which they had been seconded.

sample, who entered the Course and did not qualify, and also those to whom was awarded a mark of distinction. It seemed that from these, especially from the former group, we might hope to learn indirectly, and so with the least distortion, about the combination of qualities regarded as essential for psychiatric social work. The addition of these two groups brought the number of subjects studied up to ninety-three.

By the courtesy of the Director of the London School of Economics we were allowed to make use of the records of selection and training kept for each student of the London Mental Health Course, of which the reports of selection interviewers and of tutors and supervisors were especially important for our purpose. In the sense that these records were made without anticipation of the kind of questions we should want to ask of them, they may be regarded as historical documents. This is true even though we ourselves were the writers of a considerable part of them and were able to supplement written records from our unrecorded memories and impressions. For the third phase, that of practice, records failed us and we had to turn to other methods.

We had in any case always meant to add to the material through personal interviews. This has often been described as the characteristic 'tool' of the social worker; it would be something with which both our subjects and ourselves should be very familiar and was the obvious method to use for our study. We decided to base the interview on a scheme of questions, by means of which we hoped to hear from the subjects about their experiences in applying for training and being selected, in the training itself and in practising their profession. We particularly wanted to know how far they considered that the training had prepared them for the kind of work which they were in fact called upon to do and how, in the course of their career, they had increased their professional understanding and skill. In personal interviews this questionnaire was used with great flexibility; it was simply an indication of the ground we wanted to cover. In the seventeen cases where a personal interview could not be arranged, this scheme was used as a questionnaire to be completed in writing. A few subjects were probably able to express themselves more freely in this less personal way, but on the whole the material from the interviews was incomparably the fuller and more valuable. The interviews had a very individual stamp; one subject would have almost forgotten her experiences at selection, but would have much to say about being a student, while the interest of another would be centred in the way her career had shaped itself after training.

During the personal interviews both parties must have had in mind the fact that the two people undertaking the study had played a considerable part in the training. Criticism of this was likely to imply some criticism of one or both of us. To claim complete objectivity on either side would indeed be absurd, but, within the limits of the situation and as far as lay in their power, the majority of the subjects seemed to co-operate in the study with commendable frankness and absence of self-concern, even those who, on their own showing, had put up deliberate defences at their selection interviews. One sign of this spirit was the readiness with which, almost without exception, subjects whom it seemed reasonable to ask gave us permission to approach two persons, one a psychiatrist and one not medically trained, who were, or had been, closely associated with their work. From these 'referees' we hoped to obtain an assessment of the subject's achievement in the practice of her profession, which we could compare with assessments made at selection and during training. We also framed questions which would draw out the referees' ideas of what psychiatric social work was, the special contribution which it could make in hospital or clinic or in the community and how the work might be improved and put to better use. The willingness of referees to cooperate in our inquiry was at least as striking as that of the subjects. Some of them, the psychiatrists in particular, seemed glad to have an opportunity to express their views about psychiatric social work and workers. Taken together their answers showed what various conceptions existed of the nature of this work and the service it could render, and how differently the emphasis was often placed by psychiatrists and psychiatric social workers upon the various aspects of the latter's profession.

When our inquiry was completed, we found ourselves with a considerable body of material on a wide range of subjects which, even after allowing for the fact that our interest in the people concerned might have led us to over-estimate its value, seemed to us of some importance. With regard to its reliability, most of the subjects entered training ten years or more before the date of our study and memories, particularly of experiences at selection, had in some cases become blurred. Often this might be attributed merely to the passage of time. When however a subject, whose suitability had been so much in doubt that, in the course of two applications, she had been put through the ordeal of six interviews, told us that, strange as it might seem, she had not been interviewed at all (and repeated her statement when the matter was taken up with her again), we were forced to recognize a forgetting of a different kind. The possibility of distortions of memory from various causes must be kept in mind in regard to all those accounts of experiences, our own included, on which this book is largely founded, as must the possibility that opinions, attributed to an early stage, have been moulded by later experience.

The material proved difficult to handle. The confidential nature of some of the personal communications inevitably raised problems. It was easy to present without danger of identification a single experience at one stage of a subject's career, but such glimpses were of restricted interest and might easily prove misleading. What would have brought the material to life would have been to have given something in the nature of a full 'case history', and this was just what it was impossible for us to give. There were, moreover, difficulties more fundamental than this. The problem of combining an impersonal with a personal approach was even greater than we had foreseen. Material from what we may call contemporary records had to be related with material specially obtained for the study through interview and written questionnaire and again with our own memories and impressions and with knowledge which had come to us in ways which we could not always trace. And through it all ran our own personal involvement in what we were trying to examine. Moreover, as we were very much aware, our miniature study, while trying to capture experiences and impressions and hold them still in order to examine them, was in fact dealing with a profession which was in constant process of change and itself could only be understood against a social background which was no less in motion.

We attempted at first to make this book a report of a particular study of a particular sample of people, drawing upon our own experience to supplement and correct it. If we had produced such a monograph we should have hoped to have made detailed references to relevant studies.[1] Events made a thorough study of the literature impracticable and a number of considerations led us to revise our method. The basis of the book has come to be our

[1] Throughout this study we have been greatly indebted not only to American literature, but to personal experience of training and services in the United States of America.

personal experience and the direct knowledge and impressions which have come to us over the years from our association with the London Mental Health Course. This seemed at first sight a poor return for all the help we had received from subjects and referees of the special study, who had been so generous with their time and interest. Looking back however we no longer regard this as wasted. As we have worked over the material during a period of more than two years, it has become very much part of ourselves. Indeed we can now look upon the special study as just that further experience by which our own experience as members of a training staff needed to be enlarged before it could be made serviceable to others.

Time has been lost, and some of the questions to which we earlier gave a great deal of attention do not seem as important as they did or very relevant to the present situation. We should like to think that a process of natural selection has been at work. In that case it is reasonable to believe that some of the questions which now stand out as important, though approached through our own experience of a small profession, have an application beyond its borders and, compared with those which first attracted us, are less at the mercy of time.

CHAPTER II

ORIGINS AND GROWTH

i

IN the summer of 1937 a group of some twenty students, of varying age and experience, had nearly reached the end of a year's professional training. Many were looking rather anxiously into the future, and not without cause. Some had given up posts in which they had been well established to train for a kind of work about which their knowledge was very limited and for which it was unusually hard for them to judge their own fitness in advance. For the older of them particularly the decision to become students again had needed courage. It is true that the supply of workers with the qualification at which they were aiming was small; only about a hundred had been trained in Great Britain up to this date and not all of these were to be regarded as competitors in employment. But the demand up to now had been small also and what it would be in the future no one could foresee. The year before, when a certain local authority had advertised for someone with this qualification, the students nearing the end of their training are said to have applied in a body. The position was not very different in 1937. The professional association concerned had made itself responsible for circulating notices of vacancies for which the qualification was required. In this year it circulated just twenty posts.

Ten years later, in 1947, forty students of the same course were nearing the end of the training and, like their predecessors, were scanning the field of employment. When they applied for admission, they had probably been more aware than the candidates of 1937 of the nature of the training and the work to which it would give them access. The situation had indeed changed remarkably within the decade. Not only were the numbers doubled in this particular course; two similar courses were now established. The most striking change, however, was not in supply but in demand. In May 1947 the professional association circulated a list of vacancies which up to then had remained unfilled. Some of them had been advertised more than once and there were others, not on the list, of which the advertisements had lapsed because they had met with no response. The number of vacant posts was now well over eighty. On paper at least the possibilities for the newly qualified had been almost disconcertingly enlarged. It was a far cry indeed from the days when the whole body of students swooped upon a single vacancy.

During the intervening ten years the professional association had extended its activities and increased in standing. It had formulated its policies in various connexions, was represented on other bodies dealing with common problems and was occasionally consulted by Government departments on special issues. One of its concerns was the conditions of work of its members and, in stepping out in 1947 into the field of employment, the newly qualified might reckon on its support as something not to be despised. Yet it is questionable whether the way of these fortunate students was really much smoother than the way of those who had emerged from training ten years before. In the beginning the Mental Health Course had been organized to equip its students for purposes which were comparatively clearly defined; the types of posts which most of those who qualified were likely to enter were known in advance. By 1947 however demands were coming in from many directions; the boundaries of their field had become precise less and it was increasingly evident that the exact nature of this service was by no means easy to determine. This in itself would have mattered less but for the uneasiness to which it gave rise among those who had passed through the training. While some were content to leave their professional rôle unidentified, and indeed mistrusted attempts to define it too closely, there seemed to be a growing distress among others over what they felt as a formlessness and a lack of direction in what they were professing to do. This, as they saw it, not only placed them at a disadvantage in their dealings with other professions but undermined their confidence in a more intimate sense. Comparatively free from the bread and butter anxieties which had faced their counterparts in 1937, the students who were about to enter employment in 1947 were probably more aware than these of difficulties which belonged to the essential nature of their calling. The fact that they could exercise choice in seeking their first posts did not necessarily lead to confidence.

It is this comparatively small, self-questioning body, bearing the cumbersome but expressive name of psychiatric social workers, which is the subject of this book. We do not propose to write a methodical history of psychiatric social work even in Great Britain, much less of the whole movement of social work out of which it has arisen.[1] To render the questions which we want to consider intelligible it is necessary, however, to understand something of the movements and converging tendencies which have played a part in making this work what it is. It is with these that the present chapter is concerned.

Psychiatric social work has its roots, as the title suggests, in social work, that wide field out of which, from time to time, special shapes appear (such as medical social work or child care), bearing the stamp of the phase at which they became particularized and developing each in its characteristic way. That psychiatric social work was a comparatively late arrival does not mean that its short life has been a simple one. It is, on the contrary, the number of tendencies and movements which converge in it that give it its special nature and has made it difficult to identify. The American Association of Psychiatric Social Workers defines psychiatric social work as 'social work undertaken in direct and responsible working relation with psychiatry.'[2] This definition possesses various merits; it emphasizes the profession's rootedness in social work and indicates that while it has here been drawn within the orbit of psychiatry it retains its own professional responsibility. What the definition does not suggest is the element of reciprocity between social work and psychiatry, the need of each profession for what the other has to give, which forms what might be called the prehistory of this new profession.

The relation of psychiatric social work to general social work may be compared with that of psychiatry to general medicine. The psychiatrist is primarily a medically trained person, though he may have borrowed liberally from other disciplines, such as psychology or psycho-analysis. The special perceptiveness which comes of cumulative experience in general medicine, on which is based that clinical 'intuition' generally acknowledged to be an important element in the art of healing, remains as part of

[1] Attention is drawn to a recently published book on social case-work in this country—Morris, Cherry (ed.): *Social Case-work in Great Britain*, Faber, London, 1950.

[2] For an account of the discussions leading to earlier definitions, see French, L. M.: *Psychiatric Social Work*, Commonwealth Fund, New York, 1940, *passim*.

his equipment when he turns to the treatment of the mentally ill. In somewhat the same way the social worker with special training for psychiatric social service brings to her new calling something corresponding to the physician's perceptiveness, by reason of the fact that she has been accustomed to think and to act in relation to the 'body social', as he in relation to the human organism, body and mind. However far the reality falls short of the ideal, there exists among experienced social workers, besides actual knowledge about the structure, functioning and ills of society which it is the part of the social sciences to study and formulate, a perceptiveness in relation to the 'body social' which may be regarded as characteristic of their profession. The single term 'psychiatry' itself implies the original discipline of medicine upon which the specialization is based and within whose field it unquestionably remains. The position of psychiatric social work is more complicated. This is illustrated by the fact that it is sometimes spoken of as ancillary to psychiatry and that this, even if unacceptable, is yet a comprehensible way of regarding it. To substitute a single-barrelled title for 'psychiatric social work' would be a misleading simplification, failing to suggest, as the present name does, how it arose and what it is.

It may be useful to imagine a social case-worker in the second decade of this century, working in some agency which tries to meet certain needs of people in social difficulties. We may think of these as in financial distress, badly housed, or requiring some surgical appliance beyond their means. The reason which brings them to the agency, the reason at least of which they are aware, is usually a practical one. We may take as our example the social worker at her best, with a sound knowledge of the structure of the society in which she is working, the provisions which it makes for the general needs of its members and how special needs may be met. She will not only have a sense of responsibility for the welfare of those who come to her but will frankly enjoy people, all sorts of them, their variety and the unexpected anomalies which they reveal. As time goes on, being an observant person of open heart and mind, she will amass much knowledge of how people act and apparently feel in certain situations and how they enter into relations with one another. Her work, even if it is based on practical needs, will constantly call for the application of this kind of accumulated knowledge and she will find that, through experience, she has learnt to deal confidently with most of the demands made upon her as a professional social worker. If she is also a person of quick intuition, her understanding will have helped her to meet the emotional needs of many of the distressed people who come to her.

The importance of this kind of insight and skill has long been recognized. The character of the client and the relationship built up between him and the social worker were, of course, clearly recognized by such pioneers as Elizabeth Fry and Octavia Hill as central to all their attempts to help individuals. This recognition has never been lost among social workers, even though it may not have been subjected to very careful thinking. Yet a social worker such as we have described will often have felt baffled about the way people behave, so obviously against their own interests, and about how they seem to feel. She will have become aware of her own ignorance and her helplessness in face of the habitual behaviour of some of them and the occasional behaviour of others, people whom she thought she knew inside out but who have suddenly allowed her to catch a glimpse of depths she cannot plumb. If she has behind her a course of training in social science it is unlikely that it will have gone far in preparing her for this, and her experience will have shown her that, within the field of social work, there is no body of knowledge which meets her needs. If anything of the kind were to become available to her from outside her own field she would be admirably ready to make use of it and, with her experience of how ordinary people behave in their natural surroundings in the community, would have something valuable to contribute in her turn. Some social workers after the first world war were indeed looking eagerly to psychology, particularly psychology as applied to mental difficulties, for the help they needed. This is reflected in the *Charity Organization Review*[1] particularly in the articles by the editor on the literature in this field.

During this period, things were in fact happening in adjacent fields which were to concern social workers very closely. In general one might say that there was a breaking down of self-sufficiency, a recognition of needs which could not be self-supplied. The history of psychological medicine or of the mental health movement, with its development of what has come to be so unattractively termed a 'multi-disciplined approach', is not within our scope, though none of it is irrelevant to our subject. We can only refer to a few salient events and tendencies and then narrow our attention to the

[1] See Burt, C.: 'Psychology and Social Work', *Charity Organization Review*, xliii, 1918, pp. 4–19, 51–60.

sequence which led to the establishment in this country of the hybrid profession of psychiatric social work itself.

The increasing socialization of medicine turned the attention of the doctor to that field in which the social worker had built up her special experience and skill. The result of this included, but went much further than, the establishment of the profession of hospital almoners. Within that department of medicine which is concerned with the mentally ill, the development appears as a growing tendency on the part of the more progressive medical superintendents of mental hospitals to regard themselves as something more than benevolent custodians of persons taken out of the community for its good and their own, for whom the hospital's responsibility ends with discharge. That entity with which the social worker had always had to deal, 'the individual in his environment', influencing it and being influenced by it, began to claim the interest of the psychiatrist in a new way. The passing of the Mental Treatment Act of 1930, embodying earlier changes of attitude and introducing the voluntary patient, with his tendency to come and go (so shocking and exasperating to administrators), made it difficult for psychiatrists in mental hospitals to think of patients as socially disembodied. It is clear from the use made of the services of the Mental After-Care Association since its establishment in 1879 that it would be quite misleading to suggest that the social needs of discharged mental patients had been disregarded hitherto. Yet the increasing recognition during the years preceding the passing of the Act of the unbreakable relation between the mentally ill and the community, even while they are temporarily or permanently removed from it, brought with it implications of the greatest importance, including demands upon the medical staff of mental hospitals of a new and very exacting kind. In another sense also psychiatry was having to face the vastness and complexity of its field. The problem of those who, without being eligible for treatment in mental hospitals, were yet personally and socially handicapped through mental causes was brought home to psychiatry, as well as to the community as a whole, by the experience of the first world war and began to be seen in its true dimensions. The social worker, as we know, was aware of the problem in the person of individual clients but had so far no special equipment for dealing with it.

Of those socially handicapped through mental causes some come into conflict with the law. In the earlier years of this century, psychiatry in Great Britain was not taking a very active part in the explanation of deliquent behaviour or in the treatment of delinquents. There was little here to be compared, for instance, with the clinical work of Dr. William Healy with juvenile delinquents in the U.S.A. at that time. In the Courts, the police court missionary, untrained as a social worker but the direct predecessor of the qualified probation officer of to-day, gained ample experience of the baffling behaviour of the mentally disturbed delinquent but, like the general social worker, had no special equipment for understanding and dealing with what confronted him. Yet, from the side of research, the field of delinquency was not neglected. It is interesting to find that social workers of the London County Council Care Committees took part in the investigations which resulted in the publication of Burt's *The Young Delinquent* in 1925. The wide circulation of this work and the influence which it exerted make this association of psychologist and social workers significant.

In yet another field of psychiatry, that of mental deficiency, social workers had long been active and possessed a body of knowledge of the social problems to which the special handicap of mental defect is apt to give rise, as well as skill in dealing with them. Although, however, the Central Association for Mental Welfare, founded after the passing of the Mental Deficiency Act of 1913, co-ordinated and raised the standard of the many local voluntary associations responsible for this work, there continued to be no recognized training for social work in this field. Nevertheless from this group, awaiting, like the general social worker, a further enlightment, there had long come an impetus to service which had its effect upon social workers quite outside its own boundaries.

This period of expectation and movement which we have indicated, with its heightened sense of individual and social needs, saw the beginning of various fruitful interchanges of experience and method. Of all that was then put into circulation the discoveries of Freud, and those whose work derived from his, were incomparably the most important. Social workers were henceforth to feel, increasingly if unevenly, the influence of the main concepts of psychoanalysis. The special importance of this for social workers who were to train for work with the mentally ill and maladjusted can hardly be overstressed, and we shall return to this in later chapters.

With this new fluidity and preparedness for deeper and wider insight and for new methods of co-operation between those in adjacent fields of work, it is not surprising to find a train of significant events started, it might almost seem, by chance. For psychiatric social work the crucial action was taken by an English magistrate of a juvenile court who, travelling in U.S.A. in 1926, was greatly impressed by the work being done there in connexion with juvenile courts through child guidance methods, in which psychiatric social workers co-operated with psychiatrists and psychologists to investigate and treat the more personal problems underlying delinquency. The result was an appeal to the Commonwealth Fund of America to help to initiate similar work in Great Britain.[1] The response to this appeal covered a much wider field than that of juvenile delinquency alone, and the last few years of the nineteen twenties was a time of preparatory activities of several kinds, notably the establishment of a Child Guidance Council, to educate public opinion and to stimulate an interest in the kind of services which it was proposed to offer, and in general to hold a watching brief for the development of the child guidance movement in this country. The activity of these years is suggested by the fact that in 1926 a children's department was opened at the Tavistock Clinic and in the following year the Jewish Health Organization of Great Britain established the East London Child Guidance Clinic. Although social work was undertaken at both these clinics, there were as yet no fully trained social workers available. This was soon to be remedied. Through the generosity of the Commonwealth Fund, training was offered in U.S.A. to selected persons, in order to prepare them to forward the development of mental health work in Great Britain. Among them was a small group of social workers.

In 1929 the London Child Guidance Clinic was established with responsibility both for demonstrating the value of the new kind of service and for the training of the three classes of clinic staff. The same year saw the establishment of the London Mental Health

[1] Interesting references to these developments occur in 'An Autobiographical Sketch' by Sir Cyril Burt, published in *Occupational Psychology*, Vol. xxiii, No. 1, Jan. 1949, pp. 9–20. He tells (p. 19) of a meeting with Mrs. St. Loe Strachey, the magistrate already mentioned, who, after reading his memorandum in *The Young Deliquent* on the need for psychological clinics, came to talk over with him the possibility of enlisting American aid. He describes also how the Child Guidance Council was formed and how he became chairman of its executive committee.

Course, which was to be the first recognized training course for psychiatric social workers, with the London Child Guidance Clinic as one of its centres of practical training. Both were to be financed for a certain period by the Commonwealth Fund.

From the beginning the Course had its home in the Department of Social Science of the London School of Economics. It was thus both firmly based in social work and established in a school of the University, where a certain standard of liberal education was guaranteed. Owing its very existence to American generosity, with several of those responsible for teaching trained partly in U.S.A., it might have been expected that the London Course would have borne a markedly American stamp. In fact, while some transplanted methods were tried out in the earliest days and later given up as unsuitable for British soil, what is noteworthy is the freedom with which the Course was allowed to develop according to British views. A striking example is the fact that all students of the London Mental Health Course (and the two courses later established have followed the same line) have always been obliged, whatever type of work they plan to take up after qualification, to undergo an almost equal proportion of practical training in work with children and work with adults. This was a clear departure from American procedure at the time.

When the Mental Health Course was taking shape it found itself subjected to a number of different demands, notably from mental deficiency and delinquency where it was hoped that the new training would enable social workers to undertake case-work with more informed understanding and to make effective social recommendations. Workers in social agencies were waiting to see whether this new development would provide that enlightenment for which they had so long felt the need. Within psychiatry itself there was a difference of emphasis; on the one hand stress was laid upon the part which the social worker with psychiatric training could play in collecting the material for clinical diagnosis; on the other hand there was the ideal of the orthodox child guidance clinic, embodied in the demonstration clinic which was to be one of the training centres of the Course, where psychiatric social workers were expected to take a full and responsible part in treatment.

It was hard for those on whom fell the task of planning the training to keep an even keel with so many winds blowing. The demands made, if not mutally inconsistent, were difficult to reconcile.

It would have been only too easy for the curriculum of the Course, with its short span of about ten months, to become disastrously overcrowded and confused and indeed the influence of this convergence upon the training of so many different interests is not hard to detect, especially in the earliest years. Yet this variety of interests was both a stimulus and a guarantee. Even though the Mental Health Course, as ultimately launched, was certain to disappoint the hopes of at least some, and perhaps all, these unofficial sponsors, yet behind this interest lay a real demand. We shall try to show how psychiatric social work from time to time has had to meet external challenges to consider afresh its nature, purpose and place in the scheme of things. At this early stage it could only wait upon events. We have described the precarious prospects of those who qualified even as late as 1937. It is hard to realize, after the passage of some twenty years, how uncharted was the sea which lay before the Mental Health Course when, in 1929, it set out upon its maiden voyage.

ii

What follows is a short preliminary account of the kind of people who were in fact attracted to this training, their reasons for applying for admission, the nature of the selection process and of the training Course itself. As we have already indicated, this will refer to the London Mental Health Course alone, during the period when we had direct knowledge of it. It must not be taken to refer to the London Course as it has developed later or to the courses in Edinburgh and Manchester, although in fact much which we write of the earlier London course will have a general application.

We shall often stress the importance of variety among those admitted for training. With regard to age at entering, while from 25 to 35 was considered particularly suitable, only a lower limit (of 22) was set for those able to pay their own fees. The group entering in 1931, for instance, included a student of 22 and one of 56, and the extremes were only slightly less in 1934, when a student of 54 was balanced by one of 23. There were few sessions without the stimulus of students from overseas, some of whom had entered this country as refugees. Others came from Commonwealth countries, from Holland and Scandinavia, from Israel, India and Egypt. Women have always been greatly in the majority, so that the use of the feminine pronoun for psychiatric social workers seems a reasonable convention, yet there have been few years in which the student group did not include at least one man. Of the wide differences in experience with which students entered the Course we shall often have occasion to write.

In such a heterogeneous group motives for wishing to undertake training are likely to be varied. In a later chapter we shall consider what our study revealed in this respect; only a few comments are necessary here. Of all the statements in the list of motives given to subjects at their study interviews the one most often marked ran: 'I wanted to gain more understanding of the problems I was already meeting in my own work.' This is obviously a good starting point for such a training. Some of the subjects concerned entered the Course with the intention of returning to the work from which they had come, and some did so. Some became attracted during training to specifically psychiatric social work and on qualification sought posts, in company with those who had entered with this intention, in psychiatric clinics or hospitals.

It has to be taken into account, in considering applications for admission to the Mental Health Course, that psychiatric social work is apt to exert a special attraction upon certain people who, some knowingly and some unwittingly, hope to solve through it their personal difficulties. Some of the subjects of our study recognized that they had applied for admission with this hope. It must not of course be assumed that such candidates were unsuitable; indeed one might expect to find among them some who were particularly promising. We shall consider later this difficult problem of selection.

The generalized account which follows of how candidates were selected for the London Mental Health Course is based on the procedure in use round about 1937, the year which we made the starting point of this chapter. All candidates filled in an application form, giving the main facts of their education and career. This in itself often suggested the path by which they found their way to the Course, but further light was thrown by a covering letter, and, over a considerable period of the Course's history, by an essay on why they wished to enter it. Candidates were also required to produce a medical certificate of fitness for the training. Two referees having a knowledge of the candidate's work were asked for; no form was used but the referees were asked to deal with certain specific points. Inevitably the value of the replies varied greatly, depending upon the degree of understanding of the nature and purpose of the Mental Health Course hardly less than on knowledge of the candidate. But the importance to be attached to the reports of referees depends also upon a larger question, whether psychiatric social work is thought of as calling for qualities of a specific kind or rather for those qualities which are demanded by any form of social case-work which, in candidates with a particular trend of interest, the specialized training of the Course could develop in a certain way.

A certificate or diploma of a social science department of a university, followed by experience of some form of social casework, was the normal requirement of candidates for the Mental Health Course. The Course itself has always been recognized as only too short for introducing the student to the specialized knowledge and experience called for in her new profession, and anyone who enters ill-grounded in the fundamentals of professional social work starts at a serious disadvantage. From the beginning, however, it has been customary to admit some students in special circumstances with formal qualifications not precisely conforming to these conditions; in such cases personal qualifications are likely to be outstanding.

The personal assessment of a candidate was normally carried out through three separate interviews. One of the interviewers would be a psychiatrist associated or familiar with the training,[1] one the tutor of the Course and one a psychiatric social worker engaged in practical work. All would be in possession of information about the candidate's career.

The decision to admit or reject a candidate lay in the hands of a selection committee composed of persons concerned in the Course from various standpoints. The candidate did not appear before the Committee in person, but members were supplied with the substance of all available information about her, including the interviewers' reports. On this basis the Committee had the choice of various decisions. It could award a scholarship or admit a candidate as a fee-paying student, reject her altogether or suggest that the matter be reconsidered when she had gained some lacking qualification or further experience or had had more time to mature.

It was made plain to those candidates who were accepted that

[1] The psychiatrist's interview was not restricted, as it is now in the London Course, to cases of doubt about the candidate's suitability on grounds of mental health.

this careful personal selection did not mean that their qualification was assured, even though there was no stated probationary period. Experience has shown, however, that when an accepted student proves unsuitable, especially in regard to her capacity for case-work, a situation is apt to arise which is particularly distressing to both student and staff. It is hard to see how this can be otherwise. In stressing the importance of personality in the selection of candidates and giving it so prominent a place in training, both as a subject of study and as something to be disciplined and used responsibly in professional relations, the Course has let loose consequences which cannot be evaded, but themselves need to be studied further.

Two characteristics of the training call for special mention—the fact that academic and practical work ran concurrently for the greater part of the year, and that every student was expected, as we have already mentioned, to undergo training in work with both adults and children. It is an important consideration educationally that when all the students came together for academic studies, the minds of some were chiefly concerned with child guidance and of others with work with adults.

To understand how the academic syllabus was built up it is necessary to remember with what equipment the student, as a trained social worker concerned both with the individual and his environment, was expected to enter the Course. Assuming, on the one hand, that she had already gained experience through her previous training and employment of the way in which people behave and feel, and had tried to understand these as far as her knowledge allowed, the Course now introduced her, through lectures by experts and through reading and discussion, to the discoveries which psychology and psychiatry, including analytic concepts, have brought to bear upon the problems of human behaviour. Within the limits of a one-year course she was to be helped to a further understanding of the healthy and the sick individual, how personality normally develops and how its development comes to be disturbed, and given an introduction to clinical psychiatry. On the other hand, assuming that a student entered training with a general knowledge of social history and social structure, the Course aimed at enlarging her knowledge of the field of mental health, the history of the various developments in mental hygiene and how they are interrelated and her understanding of the social concept of mental adequacy. Against this background she was introduced to the legal and administrative provisions connected with mental illness, mental deficiency, child care and delinquency, so that, as a psychiatric social worker employed in any capacity, she could see their application to individual cases and use them discriminatingly. The Course did not offer specialized training in either mental deficiency or delinquency but, since the student might expect to be faced with individual defectives and delinquents in any work which she undertook as a psychiatric social worker, an attempt was made to introduce her to the clinical and administrative aspects of both.

In her practical training the student was treated as a responsible social worker, entrusted from the outset with her own cases, though under the supervision of members of the staff of training centres specially chosen for the purpose. It was at these centres that the greatest part of her time was spent throughout the session. The passing of students from one centre to another meant for all a considerable readjustment, both in conditions of work and in ways of thinking about mental illness. It is to be expected that members of such a heterogeneous group as we have described would feel to different degrees the strain of different parts of this full and comparatively complex course. Some might be confused by the variety of views with which they were confronted, others disturbed by being introduced to mental processes of which they had not been aware; for others the greatest strain would consist in coming into contact with persons mentally ill; others would suffer through their sense of inadequacy in face of the responsible work which they were called upon to undertake with people in emotional distress. In the chapter devoted to training we shall consider the part played by tutors and supervisors in helping students to make use of the varied experience which the Course provides.

The certificate of the Mental Health Course was granted on the advice of an examining board, which took into account the results of a written examination and reports on academic and practical work throughout the year. It was open to the Board, apart from passing or failing a student, to award a mark of distinction when her work seemed to have shown outstanding quality or unusual all-round competence. With some students it was felt that, although they had proved themselves essentially suitable for psychiatric social work, they needed a further period of practical work under some degree of supervision. In such cases this might be made a condition of being granted the certificate but more often students were merely advised to seek a post with an experienced colleague. For a few years before the war a small number of bursaries were available which met this need so far as they went, but after the war they were not revived. Although there are now more clinics and hospitals than formerly where a novice may enlarge her experience with the support and advice of her colleagues, the problem of consolidation of the formal training has not been solved. Indeed it would seem as though the march of events has never allowed it to be squarely faced, and the present urgent demand for psychiatric social workers in educational and consultant capacities in the mental health service, while it accentuates the need for training to be consolidated, does not provide the best climate in which to work out long-term plans for ensuring it.

iii

As pegs on which to hang our account of the employment of psychiatric social workers, we shall make use of three dates—1930, when the first group of students qualified in the Mental Health Course, and 1937 and 1947, the years of our original comparison. Reference will also be made to developments in later years.

We have described how behind the London Mental Health Course, when it came to be established in 1929, there lay the expectations of different groups of people, who saw it from the standpoint of the various needs and interests which they represented. We must now consider what use was in fact made of the services of the first group of students admitted to the Course.[1]

First Posts

of those qualified in the London Mental Health Course in 1930 seeking posts in Great Britain

Child guidance	*Mental hospitals or observation wards*	*Psychiatric out-patient clinics for adults*	*Clinical posts combining work with children and adults*	*Research related to psychiatry*	*Posts where Mental Health Course relevant but not required*	*Total*
3	2	1	0	1	2	9

Note: Two not seeking posts.

[1] A table is given for 1930 in spite of the small number involved for comparison with the tables for 1937 and 1947 on pp. 25, 33.

Of those seeking employment, six found posts as psychiatric social workers in clinics or hospitals, three of them with children and three with adults. These clinical posts were all in London, two of them at one of the centres of training. The remaining three workers all entered posts where they could apply what they had gained from the Course, one as assistant in a research project in mental deficiency, one in her former post as children's care organizer under the London County Council, the third in a children's home. As will become clear later, the main pattern of employment was thus laid down in the first year.

The pattern's development was somewhat uneven. The Child Guidance Council, whose work at this time was not confined to children, extended its demonstration loan service, with the result that psychiatric social workers were established in a number of mental hospitals and child guidance clinics. Occasional new demands for their services also occurred spontaneously. At this period however the demand, particularly in work with adults, was slow to develop outside London. By 1937 ten mental hospitals and five observation wards of the London County Council[1] were employing psychiatric social workers; several were also employed at the Maudsley Hospital, which had been a centre of practical training from the early days of the Course. In striking contrast, over the whole of the rest of the country the number employed at this time in work with adults was only eight. Work with children showed a similar though rather less marked concentration in London. Apart from those entering clinical posts there were to be found during the period between 1930 and 1937 a considerable number of persons who had passed through the Mental Health Course and, with the qualifications of psychiatric social workers, returned to their former posts, such as hospital almoners, family welfare workers, probation officers, organizers of children's care work and Borstal housemasters. This was the situation when the newly qualified workers of 1937 entered the field of employment.

It will be noticed in the following table that of all those employed as psychiatric social workers the great majority are attached to hospitals or clinics. In only one instance does the appointment represent the first introduction of this service. The rest point to the beginning of departments of psychiatric social work in which the

[1] Later, as more posts became available elsewhere, the scale of salary paid to psychiatric social workers by the London County Council made these posts less easy to fill.

FIRST POSTS

of those qualified in the London Mental Health Course in 1937 seeking posts in Great Britain

Child guidance	*Mental hospitals or observation wards*	*Psychiatric out-patient clinics for adults*	*Clinical posts combining work with children and adults*	*Research related to psychiatry*	*Posts where Mental Health Course relevant but not required*	*Total*
4	3	2	2	1	6	18

NOTE: Occupation of one not known

newly trained can consolidate, under experienced guidance, their short period of formal training; two of the students who in this year were considered to need this kind of experience were able to find junior posts. A considerably smaller group proceeded to posts in which their new qualification was not specifically called for. None of these, as it happens, had entered intending to return to the type of work in which they were engaged prior to their training, and all before long found their way into psychiatric social work. The fact that their first post was of a different kind seems to have been due either to special personal circumstances or to the limited number of posts available in psychiatric social work at that time. One of this group, for example, who passed from the Mental Health Course to the work of a probation officer, was to be found five years later in child guidance and has remained there up to the present time.

The year 1937 brings us within sight of war. Titmuss's *Problems of Social Policy*[1] gives the background of social planning for war-time needs against which this still very small profession, hardly ten years old, had to prove to itself and others what contribution it could make to the social services at a time of national emergency. It would not have been unreasonable to question whether it would survive the test. The few child guidance clinics established so far, which by their very nature could only serve an exceedingly small part of the population, might well have been regarded as imported luxuries and have gone down before the mass methods

[1] Titmuss, R. M.: *History of the Second World War, Problems of Social Policy*, H.M. Stationery Office, 1950.

inseparable from war-time planning. The mental hospitals had a long history behind them before the service of the psychiatric social worker had been introduced. She was an upstart in their long tradition and, in the reorganization which the Emergency Medical Service involved, might have found herself outside the mental hospital altogether or put to unspecialized uses. To an informal inquiry at the outbreak of war about the use now to be made of psychiatric social workers in mental hospitals the answer was vague; they might be useful in helping in the office or possibly in the wards, since nurses were likely to be called up.

The future of the Mental Health Course was perhaps the most uncertain of all. Its collapse might have come about through the impossibility of providing adequate training, or of securing students who both reached the standard which had been established and were free to enter the Course. One might expect too that some candidates, whose age left them freedom of choice, would not feel justified in leaving responsible jobs for the 'luxury' of a specialized training. We cannot here trace the history of the Course in war-time. It did not in fact collapse and we believe that there was profit as well as loss from the improvisations which the conditions of war-time imposed upon it. Nevertheless the reduced field of recruitment, the difficulty of carrying out even reasonably adequate selection, the extreme difficulty of ensuring conditions necessary for academic study and of providing, through emergency services, educational experiences of suitable kind and range, all these combined to make the war years a period in the Course's history which has to be regarded as abnormal.

The history of the employment of psychiatric social workers during the years of war calls for fuller treatment, since its broad results are still so markedly with us. The first effect was naturally of dislocation. In London, for instance, Government plans for the evacuation of children led to the closing down of child guidance clinics, and in the earlier period some psychiatric social workers found themselves without posts. In the meantime many were undertaking various kinds of responsibilities with displaced children. In the meetings of the Association of Psychiatric Social Workers at this time it was clear that there was a divergence of views about the functions of the psychiatric social worker in a country at war. While some members felt it all important to maintain in clinic and hospital, as far as conditions allowed, the standard of work which they had striven so hard to establish, to others this conservative attitude seemed short-sighted and rigid. Particularly to the uprooted there came from the Mental Health Emergency Committee[1] the call to pioneer. What form pioneering would take was at first not clear, but by the end of 1939 the Committee had placed psychiatric social workers in some of the Civil Defence Regions as regional representatives to explore the possibilities.

It seemed obvious that there would be a fanning out of psychiatric social workers over the country and a need to adapt accepted functions to new conditions. From discussions at meetings of the Association we had the impression that the temperaments as well as the circumstances of individual members inclined them to the conservative or the pioneering persuasion. External events were challenging the profession to examine itself and its place in the social order, but the pressure which they exerted did not conduce to clear thinking. Meanwhile, individuals were faced during this period with many problems of professional conduct which they had never encountered before in so urgent a form. One reason why psychiatric social workers found it hard to envisage where and how they could serve in the social upheaval that was to come was that, in a special sense, they belong to a profession which does not function alone. What its war-time pattern was to be could only be predicted when it was known how psychiatry itself was to be fitted into general social planning. Perhaps it would be true to say that psychiatric social workers showed no more and no less foreknowledge of the demands that would be made upon them than most of the groups of workers in the sphere of health and social welfare, and this, as Titmuss has shown, did not amount to very much. It would also be true to say that they learned and grew with their jobs.

In those hospitals and clinics where by the end of 1939 psychiatric social workers had been installed, it would seem that their work had so far established itself during the preceding decade that, in some form or another, it had come to stay. This is true in spite of the dislocation among some of the child guidance clinics and the fact that in certain hospitals some psychiatric social workers were engaged for a time in duties which were more of the

[1] Established as a war-time substitute for that amalgamation of all bodies working for mental health urged by the Feversham Committee. Report of the Feversham Committee, *The Voluntary Mental Health Services*, published by the Feversham Committee, London, 1939.

nature of hospital almoning than of the work for which they had been specially trained. In work with adults it is notable that not only were psychiatric social workers retained, but new appointments continued to occur at intervals; towards the end of the war, the demand greatly increased. In child guidance appreciation of the service which these workers had to offer grew as a result of widespread experience of the problems presented by the evacuated child.

So far we have been concerned with what may be called the orthodox use of psychiatric social work. But this still small profession was now to be subjected to new demands. First in time came the war-time social surveys. It was reasonable to expect that the training of psychiatric social workers, with its emphasis upon the interview, would have something to offer in this type of work. Moreover, from the beginning, a few of these workers had been engaged in investigation as part of psychiatric research, though openings for such work had always been few. The story of the surveys does not concern us here, but the experience which they offered to a small group of psychiatric social workers provided evidence that a specialized training, although it can be usefully adapted to a number of unforeseen situations, must carry inherent limitations. While the training of the Mental Health Course had undoubtedly developed a certain kind of skill in interviewing, concern with the effect of interviews, which is part of the professional outlook of the psychiatric social worker, was found to be not always in the best interests of the surveys themselves, however much it might further the understanding of human attitudes.

On a small scale, but no less important, was the use made of psychiatric social workers by the Admiralty, to train W.R.N.S. personnel to interview naval ratings, in order to ascertain their interests, degree of stability and level of intelligence—another recognition of the concern of the profession with the skilled use of the interview. At a later period a small number of workers were employed in resettlement units for returned prisoners of war.

The two war-time developments which involved the greatest number of workers and had the most lasting effects on the profession were the work with evacuated children and the After-Care Scheme for Ex-Service Psychiatric Casualties. Here for the first time, on a comparatively large scale, we find the psychiatric social worker not anchored on hospital or clinic but at large in the community, and exposed there to all the professional winds that blow. The complicated history of these two developments is beyond the scope of this short account. Our business is to suggest what part our profession played in them and to indicate some of the problems to which this expansion of its original sphere gave rise.

Those whose professional concern is with the meaning of behaviour and human relationships may easily under-estimate the administrative achievement of those responsible for the practical planning of war-time evacuation. They find it hard to understand the official disregard of just those things which make or mar people's living together. When children were taken out of their own environment and billeted with foster-mothers, a crop of problems arose which were not easily explicable in any terms understood by foster-mothers, billeting officers, parents or indeed the children themselves—problems which were more difficult to clear up than dirty heads and which did not respond to transfer from one billet to another and a final dumping in a hostel for the 'unbilletable'. In some cases the problems, if they were acute enough, found their way to a child guidance clinic and, in any reception area where such a clinic existed, made heavy demands on the clinic staff. There were many problems among these children which did not require the combined skill of a team of experts. The psychiatric social worker, the member of the team with the most contacts in the community, would be called upon to advise, or possibly to deal directly, with a number of difficulties which called, not for clinic treatment, but for the intervention of a social worker specially trained in the understanding of disturbed behaviour and relationships. Child guidance clinics, however, in the early days of the war were few and unevenly distributed, and touched only a fraction of the needs of the puzzled and overworked people who were trying to meet, in the reception areas, unfamiliar yet essentially normal human problems.[1] It was in response to these needs, expressed through various channels, that psychiatric social workers made their appearance in these areas, attached to no child guidance clinic and working under a variety of administrative arrangements. The supply was extremely limited and the service which resulted could not be anything but inadequate to the need as a whole. In 1942, therefore, the Ministry of Health undertook to cover the welfare problems of evacuated persons on a nation-wide basis, within which framework psychiatric social workers continued their specialized work. Apart

[1] *See* Isaacs, Susan (ed.): *Cambridge Evacuation Survey*, Methuen, 1941.

from these, the welfare officers appointed by the Ministry included organizers of children's care work, seconded by the London County Council, some of whom had qualified in the Mental Health Course and then returned to their original work.

It was not always possible to fill these highly responsible community posts with psychiatric social workers of long experience. For those who passed to such posts straight from the Mental Health Course, without clinical experience, the ordeal was a severe one. With no pattern laid down for them and exposed to the scrutiny of local social workers and officials, unless they had a real contribution to make to the tangled situations presented to them and were able to make it speedily and acceptably, they might expect to meet with a critical attitude corresponding to the force of the original need for their help. For someone who had not yet had time to build up her own professional competence the situation was full of danger. It was only too easy to attract problems beyond the scope of her training and capacity and to let herself be invested with the magical powers which others would have liked her to possess. Often it must have seemed a compelling reason for undertaking work for which her training had not equipped her that no expert help was obtainable. But it is important to remember that the evacuation scene was never a stationary one. Where first there had appeared the isolated psychiatric social worker there would sometimes later appear a child guidance service, staffed eventually, if not at once, with the psychiatrist, psychologist and social worker of the orthodox clinic team. Established at first to deal with the problems of evacuees, the service would be extended to local children and finally be taken over by the local authority. In this way, some psychiatric social workers at large returned to the orthodox clinical fold.

The contribution made by psychiatric social workers to the community care of adult patients during war-time was by no means confined to the After-Care Scheme for Ex-Service Psychiatric Casualties. Regional representative of the Provisional National Council for Mental Health (which had replaced the earlier Mental Health Emergency Committee), from the time when they were sent out to a few chosen regions at the beginning of the war, had always been concerned with community planning and education in mental health and, even when the demands of ex-service cases were at their height, had been available, as far as this work allowed, to deal with individual civilian needs. For our purpose it will be enough to give some account of the Scheme.

This, both in the nature of things and because of protracted inter-departmental negotiations, was a later development than the work with evacuated children, and it was not until early in 1944 that the Scheme was launched. A paragraph which appeared in the *Lancet*[1] in anticipation of this described how the Board of Control, in consultation with the service departments and the ministries of Health, Pensions and Labour, had committeed the organization of the Scheme to the Provisional National Council. It explained how those in charge of service psychiatric hospitals or Emergency Medical Service neurosis centres would notify the Board of Control of any patient about to be discharged from the Services who needed after-care and (a very important point) were willing to receive it. This notification was to be accompanied by a report from a trained social worker allocated by the Provisional National Council to each of the hospitals and centres, which would be passed for action to the Council. The case would be dealt with by the Council's regional social worker, who would visit the patient's home and take any necessary steps in co-operation with his doctor and with the local authority and government departments concerned. For psychiatric social workers the scheme is memorable, not only for the direct work achieved but for the opportunity it gave of exploring what part could usefully be played by a very small body of social workers with special training among other social workers and officials in the welfare services. Here was a rehearsal for the adjustments which were to be called for later under the National Health Service Act.

Like the psychiatric social workers with evacuated children, the worker in the After-Care Scheme was the object of expectation, often ill-informed, to an extent unknown to the workers in clinics or hospitals. The temptation to an after-care worker to exceed her strictly professional functions was no less than that of her counterpart working with evacuated children, and her position was more vulnerable, since the problems of adults were apt to have a larger medical component than the behaviour problems of evacuated children. In the after-care service the psychiatric social worker was working without medical direction in any way comparable to that under which she would work in a clinic or hospital.[2]

[1] *Lancet*, January 29th, 1944, p. 169.

[2] Regional representatives were encouraged by the Council to consult psychiatrists about their cases at such clinics as existed.

There was substance in the criticism that in this service she was undertaking the function of psychiatric diagnosis, in that it was she who had to decide whether to refer a patient to a psychiatrist if he was referred to her through the Scheme primarily for social work. The alternative would have been for every patient referred by a Service hospital for help under the Scheme to be sent to his nearest psychiatric out-patient clinic, where the psychiatrist would call in the help of a social worker if he considered it necessary. Apart from the undesirability of passing a patient through a psychiatric clinic if his need was regarded when he left the Service hospital or neurosis centre to be essentially social, it could not be taken for granted that a psychiatrist at such a clinic would always understand what kind of help a psychiatric social worker might be expected to render in such cases, or be prepared to call in her services. In the Scheme as it actually existed there were instances where the worker would have been only too glad to have referred a patient to a psychiatrist had she not been discouraged by the limitations of certain clinics, where no psychotherapy was attempted and the only form of treatment available was admission to the local mental hospital.

The problem was a very real one for all psychiatric social workers in regional work, who were usually well aware of the delicacy of their position. Obviously the situation was unsatisfactory and mistakes of judgment were made. Matters were greatly clarified when, a year after the war ended, a medical director was appointed to the National Association for Mental Health, together with consultant psychiatrists in every region—a plan which had been agreed upon in principle from the beginning but had proved impracticable in war-time. This provided psychiatric social workers in the regions with medical direction, the absence of which had given rise to criticism in earlier days. This was the situation when, in 1949, the scheme came to an end with the withdrawal of the grant from the Ministry of Health to the National Association for Mental Health.[1]

The end of the war naturally meant readjustments within psy-

[1] It was now for each local authority to decide whether it would make arrangements for carrying out its duties in mental health under the National Health Service Act through the Association's existing organization or undertake these duties directly. At the time of writing (1952) all local authorities except London and Middlesex have taken the latter course; on the other hand, a small number of individual psychiatric social workers are found employed in the mental health services of local authorities here and there throughout the country.

chiatric social work, but nothing comparable with the dislocation at its beginning. The work of the regional representatives of the National Association was to continue for several years, with a demand for qualified psychiatric social workers which could only partly be met. Demands for psychiatric social workers in clinical posts throughout the country had by now markedly increased, in part as a result of the direct or indirect influences of the regional representatives. The National Health Service Act of 1946 and the Children Act of two years later were to have, in varying degrees, considerable importance for the employment of psychiatric social workers; these may be left for later consideration.

We turn back now to our selected decade and for comparison with the table of first posts of those who qualified in 1937, give below a companion table of first posts in 1947.

FIRST POSTS

of those qualified in the London Mental Health Course in 1947 seeking posts in Great Britain

Child guidance	*Mental hospitals or observation wards*	*Psychiatric out-patient clinics for adults*	*Clinical posts combining work with children and adults*	*Research related to psychiatry*	*Posts where Mental Health Course relevant but not required*	*Total*
20	11	1	3	1	4	40

In face of our description of the widened field of psychiatric social work in war-time and the possibilities it opened up, the table for 1947 may seem a puzzling one. In the case of those employed in posts where the Mental Health Course was not required, it happens that a comparison with 1937 is not very profitable. Thus two organizers of children's care work are found in 1947 returning to posts from which they had been granted leave of absence to take the Course. During the war they could not have been spared for training, but before the war, for instance in 1933 or 1934, students from the same source might well have been found. What is of interest is to find that, so soon after the war, the course was again being used by social workers intending to return to their original work, as those who planned the Course had hoped it would be.

The proportion in clinical posts is markedly higher than in 1937;

the large choice of these posts in 1947 as compared with the small number in 1937 is probably the chief determining factor. The proportion of those in child guidance as compared with those in clinical posts with adults is markedly higher, yet in the following year the number of newly qualified who entered mental hospitals was more than twice the number of those who entered child guidance. We can only speculate about the reasons for these fluctuations within clinical work. A fact of greater interest is that in the year 1947, when the after-care scheme was still in existence and in need of assistant regional officers, none of the newly qualified entered community service.[1]

It would seem that in 1947 the distribution of posts among those who had just qualified is less representative of the distribution among psychiatric social workers as a whole than it was a decade earlier. By 1947 these include workers with experience of fifteen years or more, varied and extended through the circumstances of war. It is natural that some of them should be passing into types of posts not likely to be open to the newly qualified. To correct the one-sided impression of the field as a whole presented by a survey of the newly qualified, we would therefore consider the occupation at this period of all those psychiatric social workers who qualified in Great Britain and were known to have been resident there. For this we shall make use of a list,[2] issued by the Association of Psychiatric Social Workers in January 1948, which represents the situation less than six months after the time when the newly qualified of 1947 would have been entering their new posts. It will be enough to draw attention to certain of the more important trends which the list reveals.

Considerably over one-half are employed in clinical posts; the number of those in child guidance and in work with adults is very nearly equal. About one-sixth of the whole are not in salaried employment. Most of these are bringing up young families; we know that some of them are undertaking voluntary work in which their training and experience are utilized. A small but increasing number are employed full-time in the training courses, and a considerable

[1] A certain number of social workers without specialized training were appointed to work under the supervision of regional after-care officers, who were qualified psychiatric social workers; some of the former themselves later entered one of the training courses and qualified.

[2] This and the lists referred to later include psychiatric social workers trained in the courses of Edinburgh and Manchester; for our present purpose it does not seem necessary to distinguish between the three courses.

number of others, listed as engaged in clinical work, are taking part in the supervision of students' training in practical work. The figures for research posts are still very low. In community service, which, as we noted, no newly qualified workers entered in the previous year, the number employed is about a quarter of that in either child guidance clinics or mental hospitals. In addition there is a small group of those who work as psychiatric social workers in non-psychiatric organizations, such as the prison service, or an organization for the care of children. Further still from the centre, taking this to be the clinical post, we come to a group, considerably larger than the last, where the qualification of psychiatric social work is not actually demanded, however relevant it may be to the work done. These include the group of those who have returned after training to their original form of social work and, more notably, a very small number who have taken up posts as children's officers under the Children Act of 1948.

When we turn to a comparable list for January 1949 we note no dramatic shift. The proportion of those in clinical posts remains the same and the numbers of those concerned with adults and children remain almost level. The proportion engaged in research has increased. In the work outside clinics and hospitals significant, if small, changes can be detected. In the year 1949 the fate of the After-Care Scheme of the National Association for Mental Health was in the balance and could offer no security of employment to its regional workers. As would be expected our list shows a reduction of psychiatric social workers employed by the Association, and here and there psychiatric social workers appear in the health departments of local authorities. At present no coherent pattern can be seen. While the National Association had seen the country as a whole, and, as far as personnel allowed, had tried to cover it, the picture in 1949 is an oddly scattered one. A psychiatric social worker is working for a local authority in Devon, Manchester, Kendal and so on. Perhaps in these isolated strongholds a high standard of psychiatric social work in community service may be built up, which will extend its influence beyond local boundaries. In the present extreme shortage of psychiatric social workers this situation represents an alternative to the spreading of their services too thinly over larger areas; unfortunately there is no guarantee that each worker is placed, in the interests of the whole field, in the best possible position.

The list for 1949 also shows an increase in the number of

psychiatric social workers, still a very small band, who (after a period in clinic or hospital) have passed over to work of a more preventive kind, lying outside the field of mental health in its narrower sense. The most noteworthy developments are those dependent upon the Children Act. While in the list for 1948 we found a few psychiatric social workers employed as children's officers under the Act, the list of the following year shows not only that the number of these has slightly increased, but also that psychiatric social workers are engaged as tutors to university courses in child care.[1]

In this far from exhaustive account of the development of the employment of psychiatric social workers will be found the background to most of the questions which occupy us in subsequent chapters. Too much attention may appear to have been paid to the war years, yet their importance can hardly be exaggerated in a profession which, when war came, was still so tentative in its search for the ways in which it could best meet the community's needs. It is presumably true of any profession that its own development depends upon a balance between some inner necessity and the demands made upon it by the community, certain of whose needs it professes to be able to serve. If there has been some tendency among psychiatric social workers, as one of the critics whom we quote in a later chapter implies, to over-emphasize the first of these, it would seem that the community is exerting an increasing pressure, which makes it more and more difficult to forget the profession's wider obligations.

We cannot take for granted that psychiatric social work will keep indefinitely the contours which it has at the present time. Movements from within, represented by a certain restlessness which we detected in some of those whom we interviewed in the course of our special study, may drive more psychiatric social workers to service outside the field of mental health. On the other hand, the increasing responsibilities which they are called upon to assume within the mental health service of the National Health Service Act may hold within this field able and experienced workers who might otherwise have sought employment outside. The appearance of the Mackintosh Report[2] has emphasized the importance and delicacy of the task awaiting them there.

[1] Two trends, leading away from posts in psychiatric social work in the stricter sense, are considered in Chapter IX. See also Appendix I, pp. 252–3.

[2] Ministry of Health: *Report of the Committee on Social Workers in the Mental Health Services*, H.M. Stationery Office, 1951.

CHAPTER III

THREE EXAMPLES OF CASE-WORK

THIS chapter stands apart from the rest. It is meant for readers who are not familiar with the work which is the subject of the book. These brief studies of case-work do not profess to give a systematic account of diagnosis and treatment and it is not expected that they will add to the knowledge of those who are habitually engaged in this work. All we have tried to do is to illustrate a few of the kinds of case-work which psychiatric social workers undertake. For two of these cases we are indebted to past students, while with the third case one of us has been in touch over a period of eighteen years. It is to be remembered that all three are presented from a social worker's standpoint, which naturally differs somewhat from that of both psychiatrist and client.

Of the three studies the first concentrates upon what happens in the social worker's part in a case, in this instance work with the mother of a child being treated at a child guidance clinic. This is in keeping with the conditions of work in such clinics, where, to draw a very broad distinction, there is more opportunity than in work with adult patients for observing processes in slow motion. Such a case does not lend itself to the summarizing method used in the second and third. The writer of this case study has therefore aimed at showing some of the most significant things that happened between the mother and herself at the outset of the child's treatment. This necessarily gives the study a tentative and indecisive air, but this is true to fact; part of the value of the method of presentation chosen lies in its faithfully reflecting how the social worker feels her way.

The second case, with its louder and wider repercussions, and the variety of people with whom the psychiatric social worker is involved, presents a strong contrast. It would seem to demand such different qualities from the social worker that one might reasonably ask what it can be that unites these two types of work in a common profession; we hope that this is answered by the book as a whole. Such a turbulent case as this is not uncommon in the experience of workers with adult patients, who however are likely to be engaged concurrently on other cases where the contrast with work in child guidance is not so great. This case illustrates the difficulty of working at the same time with a patient and with persons who form his environment, and the social implications of mental disorder. To the reader these may seem to overshadow the social worker's therapeutic rôle. The writer is herself aware of the reader's difficulty. Her aims are clearly stated (pp. 46–7), but only someone within the stream of the case's development could assess how far her efforts were justified. And the time for assessment is not yet. The case should serve to dispel any idea that the difference between psychiatric social work in child guidance and with adults is one of profundity and superficiality. These are not determined by length of treatment or the particular methods pursued. Depths may be touched in a single interview or evaded in treatment of indefinte length.

The third case calls for little comment here. That the patient was an adolescent when the case opened makes it a bridge between the first two and gives rise to questions not inherent in either of them. A great part of its interest lies in the length of time over which it could be observed, so that it was possible to watch the emergence of quite unpredictable circumstances and the use which the patient made of them, partly as a result (one likes to think) of the help which she had received at the time when her life seemed in danger of reaching a deadlock.

NOTE.—The usual precautions have been taken against identification.

CASE I

FROM A CHILD GUIDANCE CLINIC

The relationship between parents who bring their children to a child guidance clinic and the psychiatric social worker evolves in very different ways according to the parents' wishes and needs and the social worker's capacity to meet them and understand them. Even when the parents' desire for their children to have treatment cannot be doubted, it may yet not be at all clear how far they are aware of their own rôle in the child's development, and how far they are ready to go in trying to understand it. It is essential therefore to bear in mind both the anxiety and guilt which the child's behaviour or symptoms may be arousing in the parents and to meet their need to build up a relationship in which some of these underlying feelings can be expressed and resolved. At the same time it is important to respect the limitations which parents themselves impose on the relationship.

The following is an account of the first few interviews with a mother who had very mixed feelings both about bringing her child for treatment and the extent to which she was prepared to co-operate. They illustrate the interaction of the mother's and child's problems and the mother's need to gain understanding of her own difficulties in order to deal with the child.

Susan West was an only child of eleven years who was referred for incontinence of faeces. This symptom, then occurring almost daily, had started about three months before she came to the clinic. The parents had been separated from the time of Susan's birth and she had been brought up by her mother, who had to go out to work. The father visited wife and child fairly frequently but took no financial responsibility.

The psychiatrist saw the child first to make a diagnosis. Susan was an overtly friendly child who made an easy superficial contact. She gave the impression of having strong emotions which she was unable to express because of severe anxieties, shown in her dreams. The symptom was a bodily sign of her conflict and symbolized an attempt to rid herself of feelings which, otherwise expressed, would bring serious consequences in their train.

During the waiting period for treatment, a man exposed himself to Susan and 'interfered' with her.

For most children treatment does not concern itself with direct discussion of the problem, but seeks to provide the child with an opportunity to develop a special kind of relationship with the psychiatrist. This so-called 'transference' relationship makes it possible for the child to 'live through' and so resolve his fears and anxieties; in consequence the psychiatrist's contribution is largely determined by the child's direct response to him, or by those reflected in play and fantasy. Susan came with a sense of guilt and anxiety about her body and its functions. These attitudes had been increased by her experience, which had also added to her fear of and curiosity about men. Treatment therefore aimed at providing her with an opportunity to resolve these fears through her relationship with the psychiatrist. In her case the initial stages of treatment aroused a strong emotional response.

In the first interview between Mrs. West and the social worker the impression was that Mrs. West was dealing in an intelligent way with Susan's soiling and her reactions to the sexual assault. At the same time her manner was extremely tense and it seemed clear that her feelings were at variance with her intellectual approach. She wanted Susan to have treatment, since she was most anxious that she should be given every opportunity to be cured of her symptom; at the same time she separated herself from the problem and did not reveal her personal feelings. For example, she gave unasked a brief picture of the family background and the facts about her separation, but gave no indication of her attitude towards it. She emphasized the material difficulties of cramped living conditions as one of the main causes of Susan's troubles. This concentration on facts and exclusion of feeling created an impersonal atmosphere which hampered the social worker in conveying to Mrs. West the nature of the treatment and the need for her to co-operate. She could not, she said, get time off work to bring Susan to the clinic herself and suggested that she should come and see the social worker about once a month in her lunch hour. In agreeing to this the social worker was accepting Mrs. West's own assessment of how little she felt that she could co-operate in treatment; at the same time she made it clear that such an arrangement was provisional and could be changed.

The second interview was of a very fleeting nature and confirmed the impression that Mrs. West was avoiding and afraid of becoming involved in her daughter's problems. She arrived unexpectedly to tell the social worker that Susan was showing very mixed feelings about coming to the clinic, sometimes refusing quite violently, saying that the doctor was 'rude'. Having made this statement Mrs. West wanted to leave and only stayed because she was asked to do so. In the ensuing discussion her manner indicated clearly how anxious she felt. She kept her anxiety at bay, however, by finding explanations for the events which had aroused it. For example, when Susan's resentment towards the psychiatrist was enlarged upon Mrs. West avoided expressing her fears about this by giving an explanation, viz., that Susan's behaviour towards him expressed her attitude towards the man who had exposed himself to her. Again she expressed a doubt whether a male psychiatrist could help Susan to get the 'right attitude' to sex. But when she was encouraged to develop this and so give vent to her own attitude towards sex, she immediately retracted, saying that she supposed Susan needed to make a relationship with a man, since she saw so little of her own father. She did enlarge on her desire for Susan to make a happy marriage and discussed the sex information which she had given her, then hurried away. In this interview, therefore, Mrs. West had again felt unable to release any personal feelings which the difficulties had aroused, and the relationship with the social worker remained superficial.

The third interview was at the social worker's request, after about a month had elapsed. Mrs. West arrived in an acutely anxious state, suggesting in the first few minutes that Susan should 'have a rest from treatment'. She then went on to describe Susan's interest in sex differences and sex play, about which she was very worried, and was full of questions as to the 'right way' of handling the situation. Almost the whole interview centred in these points. Mrs. West's anxiety about her own inadequacy and fear that Susan's behaviour was abnormal came out fairly clearly, but the social worker did not feel that the relationship warranted an attempt to approach these attitudes except indirectly. Rather than getting down to giving advice about the 'right' methods of handling, she encouraged Mrs. West to talk about her own methods of dealing with the behaviour, and discussed this in relation to Susan's development and experience, in this way shifting the emphasis from Mrs. West's explanations and handling on to Susan's need to express her fantasy. Finally, near the end of the interview, after having enlarged upon her own views, Mrs. West gained sufficient confidence to express openly the feeling that perhaps she was directly to blame for Susan's difficulties, limiting her responsibility mainly to Susan's failure at school. She herself had not been allowed to take up the scholarship which she had won and had made up her mind that Susan should be given every educational advantage; she now had the feeling that it was her desires which were in some way preventing Susan from making progress and said 'perhaps I am the nigger in the wood pile'. Having partially divulged her sense of responsibility, she said that she would like to come again the following week.

At the fourth interview Mrs. West started expressing doubts about treatment. She put forward the idea that the emphasis should be on the 'good side of life', whereas bringing Susan to the clinic was stressing the symptom. She felt, however, that her own approach had failed. Having talked about her ideals she expressed her despair at the way in which she had not been able to live up to them. She described how angry she got with her husband and the quarrels they had, although, when he was not there, she tried to build him up as a good and gifted person. She blamed herself for giving Susan such a bad example of married life and felt that it would make it impossible for her to enjoy satisfactory relationships later. At this point the social worker asked Mrs. West about her own experience, which she poured out with considerable feeling. She had had an unhappy childhood with an 'over-sexed' father, who was violent at times. She left home when she was seventeen years and married young. She considered that the first few years of her marriage were happy; she and her husband shared intellectual interests and he was 'kind and considerate'. She then wanted a child, and, when her husband disagreed, 'tricked' him into it. From the time of Susan's birth he refused to live with her, blaming her for the child and accusing her of being sexually demanding. For a time she hoped he would change his mind but slowly gave up expecting this, and could not get over her resentment at the way in which he refused to share responsibility with her. When Mrs. West again blamed herself for her attitude to her husband, the social worker avoided becoming aligned with this self-accusing attitude and queried both the possibility and the value of creating a 'good' but unreal façade for Susan. In discussing this Mrs. West described other relationships, from which it appeared that she always took the responsibility for keeping things 'good', however aggressive and difficult she felt that other people were; this attitude imposed a constant sense of strain. She left the interview in a friendly way, saying that she would be coming the following week.

The next day Susan had a treatment session in which she seemed driven to develop her fantasies about men's bodies, particularly about the act of mating in relation to herself. The psychiatrist did not find it possible to allay all the anxiety which this aroused within the one session.

Mrs. West telephoned the next morning, insisting that she must see the social worker the same day. When she arrived she made an open, angry attack on the clinic, demanding to know what the psychiatrist had been saying to Susan. It appeared that she had been worried and excitable the night before and had asked for an explanation of the sexual act, which Mrs. West had given. In meeting Mrs. West's anger the social worker showed her realization of the anxiety which the situation had aroused, suggesting that Mrs.

West's attack probably resulted from her feeling that she had been burdened with another responsibility of the same pattern as the one which appeared in all her relationships, viz., of trying to keep things 'good' against impossible odds. When the social worker made this attempt to understand Mrs. West's attitude rather than refuting the charges against the psychiatrist, Mrs. West relaxed and started to discuss the nature of treatment more fully. In doing so she showed a greater ability to tolerate Susan's need to express her fantasies, and less fear and doubt about her ability to cope with them. She went on to say that previously she had had the feeling that she was being 'kept out' of Susan's treatment, but that she realized now how necessary a part she had to play. When the social worker agreed that her outburst had led the way to a better understanding, Mrs. West said that she felt that it was not 'too late' to do things differently, and confirmed her desire to develop the relationship with the social worker by making an arrangement to come to the clinic weekly.

It should be mentioned here that during this initial stage of treatment, with the release of fantasy and feeling, including hostility towards the psychiatrist, Susan's soiling had improved considerably, although of course the major part of the work in resolving her conflicts still remained to be done.

Although these first five interviews had only just touched on Mrs. West's personal difficulties, they do illustrate how, through the growth of the relationship with the social worker, Mrs. West was enabled to play a part in treatment on a deeper level than mere acquiescence in Susan's attendances. When she first came to the clinic she was imbued with a sense of failure and a deep mistrust of her own feelings. This mistrust, and the consequent sense of strain in all her relationships, determined her approach to the social worker. Her attitude, which had contributed to Susan's difficulties, had also made it impossible for her to deal either with Susan's negative attitude towards the psychiatrist (which existed side by side with more positive feelings) or her expressions of curiosity about sex, except on a purely intellectual level which thinly disguised her anxiety and failed to reassure Susan. Mrs. West's sense of inadequacy in face of Susan's behaviour finally led her to give expression to some of her doubts and fears and some of the experiences which had helped to create her attitude. Her ability to express her aggression in the fifth interview, in place of withdrawing Susan from treatment altogether, depended upon the relationship which had been established with the social worker. It was only when Mrs. West found that she was still accepted in spite of her aggression, thus experiencing the possibility of change in the past pattern of her relationships, that she came to feel that the situation was not hopeless and that she had a part to play in Susan's treatment.

CASE II

FROM A MENTAL HOSPITAL

Mr. Michael Watson, a twenty-eight-year-old clerk, was admitted to a mental hospital as a voluntary patient suffering from delusions of persecution. He believed, wrongly, that he was being accused at work of writing obscene remarks on official forms, and at times feared that the supposed accusations were true. He was an intelligent, studious young man, interested in poetry and music; capable of warm feelings, but rather solitary; unpractical in everyday matters and at times lazy, but capable of spurts of energy, intellectual honesty and moral courage.

The social worker's first contact was with Mr. Watson's sister, who was sent to her by the doctor to give a 'social history', before there had been an opportunity to obtain the patient's consent for this. To have the patient's consent before taking a history is important, not only out of respect to his confidence but because the interview in which consent is asked, being focused on the patient's present family situation as his first interview with the psychiatrist is unlikely to be, will enable him to bring his family tensions into the open and sometimes to see them with a little detachment. When he decides to trust the social worker to see his family, a beginning has already been made in the social treatment. In this case Mr. Watson's trust in the social worker's dealings with his family had to be built up later.

The first interview with the sister not only produced the outline history (amplified in many later interviews), but, by giving her an opportunity to display her resentment at his recent boorish behaviour and then leading her back to recall with warm affection his normal character, established a relationship in which she could turn to the social worker for help in her later difficulties and in which her fundamental loyalty to her brother could have free play.

Mr. Watson was the youngest son of a father who died just after his birth and a mother who, left a widow with five young children, had, following her confinement, a severe mental illness, which, untreated, became chronic. She remained suspicious, intensely deluded, fiercely protecting her youngest son from the many 'plots' that threatened her. He was treated as a baby, and shared his mother's bed until well on in childhood. His good intelligence won him a place in a secondary school, but his mother scented a plot in this, and stopped him from going. Though rather reserved as a boy, he was quite a leader among a small group of friends. After a period at a commercial school he started work as a clerk. Like an older brother who had earlier emigrated, he longed to get away and to escape from his mother's nagging protectiveness. The war gave him his chance. He joined the R.A.F. and trained overseas but, when nearly through his course, was disqualified from flying by a physical illness and was transferred, disappointed, to the Navy. On demobilization he returned to clerical work, did extremely well in his office, passed examinations and won promotion. He continued to live with his mother, in resentful dependence. He thought much about sex in the abstract, but could make no close friendships with girls and was preoccupied with his unrequited love for a girl whom, in fact, he scarcely knew. For some months he had worried about himself, and was reading a great deal of psychology. When he became convinced that he was accused of writing the poison pen remarks, he impetuously demanded to see a psychiatrist, declaring that he knew he was 'part mad', and could hardly wait for admission to hospital.

Just as impetuously a few weeks later, after he had begun a course of insulin coma treatment (the specific treatment for his illness) but before there had been time for improvement, he insisted on leaving. As it was considered unsafe for him to leave hospital at this stage, he had to be certified. It was the social worker's job to see the sister and other relatives, explain the reasons for certification and win their co-operation. She also had to deal with numerous financial matters arising from the certification, made more complicated by the mother's delusions which at that time centred mainly round money. She had frequent contact with the welfare officer at his office, getting his account of the patient's abilities and his behaviour at work, arranging for his job to be kept open, for payment of his salary and for transfer to another department when he should return. All this involved frequent if superficial contact with the patient.

When, after six months in hospital, he had lost his delusions but was able to remember and repudiate them and was ready to leave, these contacts led him to come spontaneously to the social worker to ask for help in planning his future. He discussed his difficulties at home, how he chafed under his mother's hovering protectiveness and how her persecutory delusions stirred up his own secret fears, though he knew them to be irrational. He felt he must break away and proposed drawing £100 of his savings and moving to the other end of the country, without address or job in prospect. He was eventually persuaded to return to his old job for the time being, apply for a transfer to another district, and go with plans properly made. This brought up his fears of returning to a job where he felt he would be known and ridiculed. Here all the preliminary work with the employer's welfare officer enabled the social worker to reassure him, and eventually he plucked up courage and returned to work. With the patient's transition from hospital to the community the rôle of the social worker changed.

From now on she worked principally with the patient himself, and the relatives, though much in the picture, were no longer the centre of it. The aim of the social worker during this period was to try to help the patient to free himself from his over-dependence on his mother and to establish himself independently in work and personal relationships, and at the same time to try to help his family to tolerate his difficult behaviour and to let him go. It is worth noting that his case was not deliberately chosen as one for intensive after-care, but became so by its own stormy development. During the after-care period the social worker was Mr. Watson's principal link with the hospital. The psychiatrist, though always informed of developments and ready to advise, saw the patient only rarely, usually when readmission on certificate seemed imminent. The aim of after-care was not only to help the patient to readjust himself to outer reality, but, at a deeper level, to stand by him in his spitirual struggle to come to terms consciously with the unconscious forces, personal and general, which disturbed him. Again and again he seemed on the point of making a decisive leap of imagination which would have landed him in safety—the act of turning to face and accept his own fears, and of giving up the defence of attributing his troubles to the conspiracies of others. But each time he misinterpreted his own need in terms of some act of physical escape in which he came to grief. To anyone reading a bald summary of his behaviour during these months it might seem incredible that there could have been any doubt about certifying him long before this was actually done, but, in the day to day unfolding of the case, each crisis seemed to be a real turning point and the full insight which followed it gave ground for the belief, shared by the doctor and the social worker, that it might be the starting point of a decisive improvement. A clinic interview which was expected to lead to certification was apt to end in the making, with the patient, of plans for some fresh venture in social readjustment.

Soon after leaving hospital Mr. Watson sent word that he was after all leaving the district to work elsewhere, but did not know where he was going. The social worker lost contact until some months later, when Mr. Watson's sister reported that he had returned and was moping at home, refusing to go to his job (which was still open for him), and that he wanted help. It appeared that he had made a half-hearted attempt at suicide, bolted without plan to the other end of the country, failed to find work or lodgings, and run through his money. Friendless, hard up and a prey to the fears of his disordered mind, he had been driven from town to town. While in London he had read in the papers of some London boys being drowned, and, at once concluding that his presence there had caused this and would continue to cause similar disasters, took the next train home. Since his return he had, on his own admission, had frequent outbursts of violence towards his mother, whose exaggerated terror of him made him feel more insecure and wild. He had been behaving in a bizarre way with knives and on one occasion chased his little niece. He was intensely distressed by his own behaviour, and asked help to get back to work and make friends; but it was a question whether he could manage this, or whether he needed immediate readmission to hospital. He could not go on as he was. His only chance was to make a break with his mother, but he had proved himself unable to work away from home. He would not return as a voluntary patient but came voluntarily to an out-patient appointment, although knowing that he might be certified. The psychiatrist, however, advised that he should return to work and go into lodgings.

For the next four months the social worker tried to steer Mr. Watson through a succession of similar crises, to help him to settle in work and in his lodgings, and to find him openings for social contacts in the psychiatric social club run for ex-patients, and in other groups where he could meet people who shared, for instance, his lively interest in poetry and music. At the same time she tried to allay his mother's exaggerated fear and her possessiveness, and supported the sister in her brave attempt to 'carry' two relatives who were mentally ill and at war with one another as well as to keep the peace with a husband impatient of her involvement. Meanwhile she was trying to remain open and loving towards her brother when he accused and suspected her, transferring to her his incompatible feelings for his mother. The sister gained confidence, even in dealing with acutely disturbed and violent behaviour, by seeing that the patient could be normal with the social worker; and Mr. Watson, though deluded and suspicious about his family, and troubled at times by fleeting suspicions of the social worker, was prepared to accept her contacts with his relatives.

After a further outburst at home he got into lodgings, settled fairly well at work, put in his notice, settled again, applied for transfer to London, withdrew his application, made a violent attack on his sister and calmed down again. He was constantly driven to peculiar actions by his feelings, which recurred in many forms throughout the case, that he carried the guilt and responsibility for all sorts of public crimes and disasters or for the misdeeds of people in his personal circle. Sometimes he reacted (as in the initial delusion about the obscene scribblings) by believing himself accused; at other times (as with the drowned boys) he accepted the guilt as his own and tried to make atonement. At times he felt himself the victim of human conspiracies, at others of 'mysterious forces far beyond my comprehension, which have been weaving a pattern round me all my life, and I never knew it'. He wrestled with his suspicions and had periods of insight. He made another very ineffective attempt at suicide, after which he appeared much steadier and free from delusions, but still determined to get away for a 'new start'. He applied to emigrate overseas but, while still awaiting the results of his medical board, was suddenly transferred to London, the long cancelled and now undesired application having at last been dealt with. He had to leave London suddenly for delusional reasons within a week, and came home to find that, contrary to everyone's expectation, he had passed his medical board for emigration. Within a few hours he had booked his passage and paid for his ticket. He had no plans, no friends at the other end and no job in prospect, and no idea of the conditions; and he wanted none. He felt a deep need to take a total leap in the dark. His sister, who understood this need, was prepared to let him go, with all the risks, and the psychiatrist, very hesitatingly, decided against interfering. But the mother, after a further row at home, took matters into her own hands and called in the duly authorized officer,[1] who had no hesitation in admitting the patient to hospital at once on a three-day order.

After a very stormy period he again left hospital, a good deal improved, but his confidence in everyone connected with the hospital had been much shaken by the manner of his admission, for he felt that he had been tricked into hospital by a plot. Previously, when he had seemed bound to be certified in the near future, the social worker had generally been able to prepare him for the possibility, and this in itself had steadied him and preserved his confidence; but on this occasion the mother had acted suddenly and without the social worker's knowledge. He was unco-operative in hospital, and mistrustful of the social worker after leaving. He at once renewed his application to emigrate, passed his medical board, and sailed in a few weeks after his discharge, this time having made rather more rational plans. He seems, however, unable to break from his dependence on his mother and at the time of writing has just returned to her, having asked her to send him the fare back to this country.[2]

The ultimate aim of the case-work—the resettlement of the patient in adult independence which at one time seemed feasible—has failed. Even so there has been for a time some strengthening of the patient's adaptation beyond his family circle and of the understanding and tolerance of his relatives. Much work with mental patients is of this nature. Risks to the community must be weighed against the patient's claims, which, unreasonable as they may seem, may hold the clue to social restoration.

CASE III

FROM A PSYCHIATRIC OUT-PATIENT CLINIC FOR ADULTS

Agnes Gifford was just under eighteen when she first attended a psychiatric out-patient clinic, referred by another hospital where she had been treated for some minor injuries, which were regarded as self-inflicted. She was brought by a sympathetic welfare officer of the firm where she worked. A gauche, immature girl, rather sullen and resistive (which indeed was not surprising since,

[1] An officer statutorily empowered to remove a person of unsound mind to a place of safety under the 'three-day order' (Section 20 of the Lunacy Act, 1890), or to initiate certification.

[2] The patient is now reported to be overseas.

between firm and hospital, she must have felt that she was brought to the clinic under duress), she did not seem altogether unfriendly and did not refuse to take part in a psychological examination. This showed an average intelligence. A social history was asked for by the doctor and a visit paid to the home, although the welfare officer had warned the social worker, on her own long experience, that it was unlikely that she would be able to establish any sincere relationship with the foster-mother with whom Agnes lived. She proved to be a woman of something over sixty, apparently a heavy drinker and deteriorated in her habits, with a kind of maliciousness which might have been a symptom of senility. Under a superficial friendliness she was obviously hostile. She described how she had taken Agnes as a foster-child at a very early age and how, when the mother almost at once ceased payments, she kept the child out of kindness. There was good reason to believe that the latter statement was untrue, but Agnes had accepted it and it had laid on her shoulders a heavy burden of obligation. Because it was felt unlikely that any better relation with the foster-mother would be established through further visits, and also because it was feared that Agnes might be made to suffer because of them, it was decided not to pursue the history-taking any further.

The account of the present situation came therefore chiefly from Agnes herself, but was corroborated in several ways as time went on. A girl of some personal refinement, she was sleeping in an unventilated and ill-kept room with an old woman of alcoholic habits, who woke her frequently during the night to attend to her, crying out with pain, of which the nature was obscure but which Agnes had been made to believe might be due to cancer. Her behaviour was unpredictable and Agnes would sometimes be turned out of the house in the evening to walk the streets for hours until the foster-mother was ready to let her in. She never knew in what mood she would find her when she returned from work. Treatment was established, more quickly than might have been expected, with an experienced psychiatrist, who gave Agnes as much time as the conditions of a busy out-patient department would allow. It was agreed that she should attend hospital in working hours without reference to the foster-mother, an arrangement which seemed unavoidable but which caused Agnes considerable distress of conscience. There was no change of psychiatrist and the only serious interruption in treatment over a period of one and a half to two years was when Agnes herself stayed away for a time, when treatment was approaching a crisis. Looking back over a period of many years, it seems clear that the self-inflicted injuries were an inarticulate call for help on the part of a patient in an intolerable situation, who gave from the first an impression of fundamental integrity which has been fully confirmed.

During the earlier stage the social work was in the hands of a student, but when she left the hospital one of the writers of this book took her place. A good relation with Agnes had been built up during the first stage, which laid the basis for all the work which followed. Contact had been kept during this period with the welfare officer, and it was possible to help her to understand more clearly the meaning of the disturbed behaviour which would show itself at work from time to time, when Agnes's treatment with the psychiatrist reached a critical point. One of several occasions on which the psychiatrist definitely called in the help of the social worker is worth mentioning. As so often happens in such a situation, Agnes had fantasies of a loving mother, in spite of the foster-mother's story that her mother had early deserted her. At a certain point in treatment Agnes became very eager to get into contact with her and the social worker was asked to try to trace her and arrange a meeting. This was done, although it was only with reluctance that the mother agreed to see her daughter, and then only in a tea-shop. The meeting proved as disillusioning as was to be expected, but seemed, as had been hoped, to have removed a barrier in treatment with the psychiatrist. The social worker gave her support throughout this disturbing experience, as a trusted person whose understanding of the situation could be taken for granted.

When the second social worker entered the case the use which Agnes made of social work took a rather different form. This change might be attributed to the different age and personality of the second worker and the conditions in which the interviews now took place. It is probable, however, that an equally important factor was the development of the patient through her treatment with the psychiatrist, so that what she was needing from the social worker had itself undergone a change. It happened that the only time when the latter was available was while she was eating a picnic lunch. Nothing could have presented a greater contrast to the formal interview with the psychiatrist, and it is possible that this helped to prevent the confusion of rôles which might have arisen when Agnes fell into the habit of coming to see the social worker regularly, straight after her psychiatric interview. We are certainly not suggesting that such a setting is desirable for psychiatric social interviews, but rather that in this case it could be used to advantage. The contents of the interviews with the psychiatrist were very rarely mentioned in the interviews with the social worker, but their effect was often indirectly apparent in the problems of day-to-day living and of personal relations which Agnes chose to discuss there. As a rule she talked easily, yet for many months would refuse any invitation to sit down during the twenty to thirty minutes interview. Occasionally she brought a friend with her, thus ensuring that on that particular day no intimate subjects were discussed. It is interesting to speculate whether these were the defences she herself erected against the informal conditions which at first might have made her uneasy. In any case this defensive period passed and Agnes found her own ways of using the interviews.

From an early stage in the case, a break with the foster-mother had been discussed between psychiatrist and social worker. There were no practical obstacles. The foster-mother was not dependent on Agnes's earnings and these were enough to support her in a hostel or lodgings. The problem lay in the sense of guilt which would certainly have overwhelmed her if she had made the break before she was psychologically prepared. Yet it was recognized that a crisis might occur suddenly and that some night, when she was once more arbitrarily locked out, she might find herself ready to leave. The social worker therefore gave Agnes her private telephone number, doing this with complete confidence that Agnes would respect her privacy in any but a genuine emergency. It was also planned in advance where she should find shelter temporarily, if she decided to leave home at short notice.

It seems characteristic of the spontaneous unrolling of this case that these carefully laid plans were never in fact used, although Agnes did leave her foster-mother and did use the worker's telephone number in an emergency. As treatment proceeded her social life broadened still further, and she came to know a young clerk, to whom she became engaged and into whose family she was accepted. This was for her, as an illegitimate child, a very important matter. Not long after the engagement her fiancé had to undergo an operation and died under the anaesthetic. The news came on a Sunday, when no help from the psychiatrist was available; it was then that she rang up the social worker and came to see her. Next day it was possible to refer her back to the psychiatrist. The break from home followed quickly, but there was now no problem of accommodation for the social worker to help to solve. It was a sign of the development of her social relations that she had come to know a young married couple at her place of work and went to live with them, an arrangement which proved a happy one.

About this time the psychiatrist left the hospital and it was decided that Agnes was now able to carry on without further psychotherapy, although it was important that she should still feel the hospital behind her. It happened that at this time the social worker would not have been able to see her frequently. This was not necessary, however, for another phase had begun. She was now ready to try out her new skill in living and the opportunities were also there to hand. After a considerable interval she wrote to the social worker to ask whether she could see her and an appointment was made. The difference between the natural and socially easy person who visited the worker now and the girl who for months had been unable to sit down in her presence was astonishing. She filled in her story since the last meeting. Soon after her fiancé's death and the break with her foster-mother, she had also changed her place of work. A friendship with a customer, while she was employed as a waitress at a tea-shop, led after a time to an engagement and again to a happy acceptance into her fiancé's family, which for generations had been associated with fairs. This point was of great importance. In this rather unusual family setting, with its tolerance combined with clear standards of conduct, the problem of how to admit her illegitimacy when faced with marriage faded away. One may say confidently that no planning or manipulating social worker could have provided this particular solution, or perhaps even envisaged it. What followed must be very briefly told. After one miscarriage a son was born, and Agnes's letters describing his development showed remarkable natural wisdom about how things look to a child, as well as an awareness of how she might use her experience of an unhappy childhood, and the insight which psychotherapy had given her, to understand and help him. Her contact with her foster-mother had been resumed some years before. It was clear that she now felt a free person and her attitude to the past was genuinely magnanimous. The foster-mother's death evidently disturbed her deeply, but she was greatly reassured at this time to find that her husband was well aware that, in spite of the psychotherapeutic help she had received, her early experiences had left her with special emotional difficulties.

This case has been chosen not as a psychiatric 'success story' but as an example of someone who was ultimately launched, through concerted psychiatric and psychiatric social treatment, into the stream of living. In a recent letter Agnes happened to revert to the period of her treatment, and her references to the help received from both psychiatrist and social worker made it clear that she had never found the situation confusing.

CHAPTER IV
SELECTION

i

Vocational selection is one of the most important modern uses of knowledge of human personality and behaviour. The right to control entrance to a profession is seldom questioned. It is however difficult to justify this limitation of individual choice unless the methods used are continually submitted to scrutiny. Reliable prediction is not the only test. The opportunity of the candidate for discovery in the course of selection has a value in itself. Rightly handled this may in a measure replace in value the liberty of choice in a 'free market'.

The following chapter is an attempt to look critically only at the methods which have been used in this particular training. We should have liked to have been able to set this against a job analysis. A study of this kind should also be compared with the significant work that has been done upon the use of standardised tests of ability and personal attitudes carried out both with individuals and with groups.[1] The fact that our material does not provide for these comparisons does not imply that they have been disregarded. In whatever way these may come to be used we think that there is a place for the more individual method of study that we have employed, for reasons which we hope will become clear.

In this chapter selection will be considered from three points of view: from that of people responsible for selection, especially for personal interviewing; from that of candidates who choose the profession of psychiatric social work, approach their selection in certain states of mind and have certain views about the selection procedure; from the general standpoint of the adequacy of the methods of selection in use as a means of prediction. We shall not attempt to consider here that urgent problem of how to attract suitable candidates.

We start at the point at which people apply for admission to

[1] Other methods of particular interest which have been used with candidates for this kind of training are the writing of autobiographical accounts, Rorschach tests, leaderless group discussions and more standardised types of interviewing.

a training course and shall take as our basis the London Mental Health Course as we knew it. The first phase of selection is general and impersonal and consists of laying down and applying those formal qualifications of education and experience which we have described in an earlier chapter. In special circumstances candidates have been admitted to training whose qualifications have not corresponded exactly with those laid down, especially when there has been good reason to think that they have a special contribution to make to the profession. There are some candidates, however, who themselves make an urgent claim to be exempted from the ordinary conditions of entry, and these will sometimes make a very different impression. Those who interview for selection have always to examine carefully this wish to be treated differently, so as to discover whether it represents a general attitude to life or is an expression of a firm conviction of a flair for psychiatric social work, unrelated to the discipline of training. In either case the candidate's suitability is open to doubt.

How a candidate regards the formal conditions laid down for admission may thus throw light upon her general attitudes, one of the most important questions in the selection of a candidate on personal grounds. This is a matter upon which reports of referees might be expected to throw light. We pointed out in Chapter II that the value of references for selection to such a training as this partly depended upon whether the work for which it prepared was or was not specific. The value of reports from tutors of social science courses and others familiar with the demands of the Mental Health Course, as well as with the qualifications of the candidates, cannot be doubted. About the reports of other referees there is less certainty; our study did not help us to form any general opinion on this point. There can be no doubt that knowledge about a candidate's previous career is important in selection for psychiatric social work, but how best to obtain this and apply it to the new situation is a difficult matter which needs, we suggest, to be further explored.

Whatever the value of referees' reports, those responsible for selection for this profession are likely to trust, to a large extent, to that process which occupies so large a place in psychiatric social work itself, the interview of one person by another. It is this means of selection which we shall now consider, from the standpoint of the interviewer. We shall not try to comment on the many features which are common to all interviews concerned with assessing personal qualities. These have been treated by R. C. Oldfield in *The Psychology of the Interview*,[1] a book which anyone with interest in this subject is likely to have read. There are, however, certain special aspects of interviewing for psychiatric social work on which something needs to be said.

In the selection procedure of the Mental Health Course as we knew it there was no set plan for dividing the ground to be covered among the different interviewers, though the position held by the three (psychiatrist, tutor and psychiatric social worker in clinical work) would inevitably influence the contents of their interviews. Thus, the tutor would take upon herself the responsibility of covering the candidate's history on the basis of the application form already sent in, while to an interviewer representing one of the training centres the work of her own centre would be a natural subject of conversation. The psychiatrist's part is discussed later in this chapter. All were equally concerned in assessing personal qualities, and this, as Oldfield points out, is done upon the basis of attitudes and abilities which the candidate is led to display.

In order to encourage a candidate to 'display her attitudes' the work on which she is engaged at the time of her application is obviously a promising subject to introduce, and one about which she is usually ready to talk. There are indeed interviews in which the candidate does not so much respond gladly to invitations to talk about her work as forces the subject upon her interviewer, and resists attempts to divert her from it. Those interviewers who are also supervisors will be reminded of students who, in the face of the new experience in which they feel at sea, cling to their achievement in former work and constantly bring round the discussion of their cases to what they have done in some earlier post. When faced with such a candidate it is for the interviewer to form a judgment about whether, through training, she is capable of freeing herself from preoccupation with the past and of gaining confidence enough to advance along new tracks.

It sometimes happens that a topic is introduced which so strongly engages the interest of a candidate, who up to this point has been chiefly concerned with the impression she is making, that she is able temporarily to forget what the interview involves for herself, so that interviewer and interviewed can talk together, as two human beings on common ground. The fact that such single-mindedness is possible, even for a short interval, in a situation so

[1] Oldfield, R. C.: *The Psychology of the Interview*, Methuen, 1941.

fraught with personal significance for the candidate, is of considerable importance. We know from experience that one of the most common reasons for not being able to make use of this training is that kind of absorption in oneself and how one appears to others which makes it impossible to enter into a client's[1] difficulties or to give oneself disinterestedly to learning. Such an interview as we have described suggests the presence of something on which those responsible for training should be able to build.

The capacity for genuine give and take is indispensable for every aspect of psychiatric social work and is a matter about which the selection interviewer should be able to form an opinion. In some cases it is obvious enough that there is some difficulty here, and the only question is whether it could be mitigated in the course of training. We remember a candidate whose manners were genuinely but excessively courteous, who appeared indeed to treat her interviewer with the greatest care. Only as the interview proceeded did it become clear that she was trying to control it by attributing to the interviewer opinions which the latter had never held, and then demolishing them. The candidate was admitted, though with a recognition of risk. When she was faced with the real demands of training it was soon apparent that she was quite unable to meet them, and that there was very little real confidence behind the façade. We remember too the impenetrable politeness and cheerfulness at selection of another candidate who later, as a student, while remaining ostensibly all too pliable in her dealings with members of the staff, showed considerable aggression in her case-work and was finally advised to withdraw. In other candidates good social poise and adroitness make it difficult to determine their real qualities in a selection interview.

Much can often be learned from asking a candidate to give an account from her own experience of some single case which brought home to her the need for such further professional training as she expects the Course to provide. This often leads to a revealing display of attitudes and throws light especially upon whether she is ready to make use of a training which is likely to involve her in personal change. A rather different group of qualities may be assessed if the interviewer should describe to the candidate a case in which she herself is interested, including the capacity to play a receptive part and to enter imaginatively into

[1] We use this term for the individual, whether patient or someone associated with him, with whom the social worker works professionally.

the experiences described to her. Talk on such professional topics will often pass on in a natural way to the candidate's personal experiences. When this happens it is likely that she will discuss these more readily, and with more understanding of how they bear upon her suitability for psychiatric social work, than if they have been introduced by means of questions early in the interview. The extraction of items of information about personal history may be a barren process, and the interviewer who undertakes it may know little about the real candidate at the end of the interview.

We shall consider later, when we come to look at selection from the standpoint of the candidate, instances of what we might call responsible reserve, in contrast to a less mature defensiveness or 'bluff'. Apart from these attitudes, there undoubtedly exists a kind of social intelligence by which the possessor anticipates the wishes and expectations of the other person and so is able to comply with them. This is not to be confused with conscious 'window-dressing'. Further exploration of the phenomena of unwitting awareness should help to clarify this particular gift. One of the subjects of our study thought of herself as possessing it, but, being an intensely self-critical person with a high standard for her own behaviour, she evidently regarded it with suspicion. In persons of less integrity and with less critical judgment such a gift is obviously dangerous, not least in the practice of psychiatric social work, though, recognized and controlled, it has a special value there. It seems likely that it came into play in the case of some of the candidates who later proved to have been overrated.

We cannot attempt to consider all the personal qualities to which interviewers pay attention. The use of the term 'qualities' is in itself misleading; no one should know better than those who have experience in this kind of selection that a particular quality or trait is only significant when seen in relation to the whole personality. A quality which might in the abstract be regarded as unfavourable can sometimes be carried by a personality which is essentially sound, and even become an asset.

Intelligence is one of the matters round which the mind of the interviewer will be constantly playing. The facts of formal qualification and, in a number of cases, the reports of tutors from social science courses will have thrown light on the candidate's general intellectual ability. The judgment which the interviewer has to make is on the candidate's present ability to learn from this particular training, and this, of course, is a very different matter. A number of qualities, such as a sense of responsibility about people, ability to co-operate with colleagues and to explain one's professional functions to others, taken for granted in professional workers whose work lies with human beings, will also be left undiscussed. We shall confine ourselves here, as far as a distinction can be drawn, to the special qualities needed for what we call the psychiatric social worker's 'chosen method', the building up of a relationship with someone in personal difficulties, within which he is helped to reach a better understanding of where his problems lie, and to discover in himself a capacity for meeting them.

The quality without which effective case-work cannot take place is the ability to make and establish a relationship with another person, which will be sincere and deep enough to bear the strains to which it will be subjected in the working out of a client's difficulties. Anyone who has been responsible for the training of students in work of this kind will remember those who have no difficulty in making quick and friendly contacts, but for whom this very facility becomes a snare. The need to keep a relation pleasant and smooth and not to risk the intrusion of anything disturbing may block any real progress in case-work. The capacity to go out to another person with warmth and spontaneity is in itself a valuable asset, and the lack of a quick response in personal relations will, on the whole, make work of this kind more difficult. With a shy and reserved worker a relationship is likely to take longer to develop. Yet given warmth of feeling and pleasure in human contacts, a pleasure which in the shy person may have a special vividness, professional relationships can be built up which bear the stresses of sustained case-work at least as well as those established by someone naturally more outgoing. This is not a simple matter to assess in a single selection interview or by one individual; perhaps there is no question in which the method of successive interviews by different persons is of greater value.

The actual helping of another person to work out a personal difficulty calls for some of the same qualities as the establishment of the relationship within which this process takes place. The essential additional quality seems to be a certain kind of imaginativeness about people.[1] In a memorandum drawn up some years

[1] We would draw attention to a paper by Roger Wilson on 'Aims and Methods of a Department of Social Studies' to which he adds A Note on 'Understanding'. He writes: 'It is a quality at once both passive and active: passive in that it receives into itself without conscious effort some part of the

ago for the use of those who interviewed for the London Mental Health Course this was defined as the 'ability to imagine truthfully the experiences of other people even though they be very different from one's own, and the readiness to accept these differences.' The memorandum goes on: 'This may be based upon an innate special ability but can probably be considerably developed through varied experience and through contact with other people who have this awareness. For some people it may to some extent be gained through reading.' Perhaps the 'beginning of wisdom' in this respect is the mere capacity to realize the range of possible experience outside one's own. Given this realization there is no end to the possibilities of developing one's 'sensibility', provided that one has the courage to keep one's imagination at the required stretch. We were interested in the opinion expressed by one of the psychiatrist referees that psychiatric social workers should be recruited from among persons of 'cultured backgrounds'; such people, he believed, have a wider range of perception and sensibility. We cannot from our own experience endorse a view which associates range of sensibility with any one social group. Nor indeed should we expect it on theoretical grounds. The difference between the amount of first-hand experience which any two individuals acquire is negligible in comparison with the variety of experience into which one is called upon to enter in any form of social case-work. Each new case should, of course, be helping to enlarge one's experience, but the solvent which makes it possible to absorb and use experience, whether direct or indirect, is that capacity to 'imagine truthfully' to which the memorandum refers. The candidate who has felt frustrated by a narrow social background has had an experience which, given this solvent, may be no less valuable to her professionally than the experience of those with greater social and cultural opportunities. In the matter of imagination individual differences count for more than differences between social groups.

It is characteristic of all social work, and perhaps to a special degree of psychiatric social work, that the worker is brought into contact with 'all sorts and conditions of men' in situations where

feelings of another person, uncritically and without distortion; active in that the whole personality of the social worker manages to convey to the client the fact that the feelings have been so received . . . I do not believe that it is a quality incapable of cultivation, by those who are prepared to soak themselves in human nature as a thing to be enjoyed and consumed, not, like beer, because it is good for you, but simply because it is enjoyable in both its bitterness and sweetness.' *Social Work*, Family Welfare Association, October 1949, p. 365.

their peculiarities tend to be underlined. Curiosity about human behaviour has its place in case-work as well as in social research, and may carry some over arid spaces, where positive enjoyment of people is at a low ebb. But we do not believe that work will prove permanently satisfying to anyone who has not a warm pleasure in people which is emotional rather than intellectual in origin. A tendency to strong likes and dislikes, on the other hand, needs to be carefully assessed. In some candidates this may be an aspect of a vivid personality, which may be well integrated and controlled. In others, however, it may represent personal difficulties of a kind liable to be especially disruptive in psychiatric social work; it will depend on the strength of the tendency and the soundness of the personality as a whole whether the former can be dealt with through the educational means which a professional training course affords.

One of the psychiatrist referees mentioned a 'reasonably happy disposition' as an important asset, and with this we certainly agree, yet when one pursues the matter further it proves elusive. A tendency to depression is not in itself an indication that a candidate is unsuitable for psychiatric social work even though, for her own sake as well as for the work's, this fact would have to be carefully weighed at selection. There is a type of cheerful disposition which may prove a handicap if, as may happen, it prevents its owner from facing the implications of what she is doing or leads to an encouraging attitude towards the client, which is more a reflection of her own mood than of the reality of the client's situation. Yet it is difficult to conceive how a worker would give to a client the kind of support which is constantly called for without a fundamental conviction that a measure of human well-being is attainable and that individuals can be helped to live more satisfying lives. There is certainly a type of unhappy person who may present herself as a candidate whom it is not difficult to recognize as someone unlikely to be content or successful in psychiatric social work. Unhappiness of this kind often contains an element of disappointed hopes and an inability to accept oneself as one is. Here we approach the view of another psychiatrist referee, that a sense of persecution is, of all attributes, the one most undesirable in a social worker (and, perhaps one should add, in anyone whose work lies with individual human beings).

The capacity for accepting another person is implicit in qualities which we have already considered, yet its importance needs to be underlined, since without it a candidate is likely to find herself ill at ease in this work. The ability to receive a client's story and to make him feel that it has been understood, to remain unperturbed by a client's behaviour, including his dependent and aggressive attitudes towards oneself, must be, if it is not a mere surface which will quickly wear thin, the expression of a much deeper acceptance of every individual's right to work out his own destiny, including the right to make his own mistakes. This capacity cannot be taken for granted in a candidate just because she is obviously intelligent, with a concern for people's welfare and an ability to establish with them a warm relationship. Indeed it is a criterion which may exclude from psychiatric social work candidates who have a great contribution to make to other forms of social welfare. Indulging ourselves in fantasy, we picture Octavia Hill as a candidate for the Mental Health Course (our imagination boggles at Florence Nightingale). We wonder whether her interviewers would have been dazzled by her qualities and by their wish to add to their profession so rare an ornament. Or would they have dared to face the fact that for certain kinds of positive personalities psychiatric social work offers not satisfaction but frustration? We comfort ourselves with the thought that the Octavia Hills of this world look after themselves and, if they should stray into the Mental Health Course, would before long pass out again undamaged on their appointed ways.

In interviewing a candidate it is important to try to discover how far she is in fact free to allow a client to be himself. It is possible to be held back from following the lead of one's client or from entering imaginatively into his experience by one's personal commitments, religious, political or whatever these may be, although, as we fully recognize, this is not their necessary result. If the interviewer is able to establish a good relationship with such a candidate, she may be able to help her to recognize the difficulties which would face her in the work for which she is applying and so to consider in advance whether her commitments and the work are compatible. There are other and not less common reasons why some people's understanding of persons and situations is limited, so that they tend to substitute a stereotyped picture for a living client. These are the unconscious commitments. It is suggested in the memorandum which we have already quoted that 'some individuals are unfitted for this work by reason of the pressure of their own feelings. This may make itself evident in a history of neurosis or may only appear in the form of attitudes towards human beings; for example, the tendency of some individuals to ally themselves with children against parents, or vice versa; or the tendency to explain all social problems in terms of a single cause, such as sex or economic deprivation.' Any hint of such rigidity which may appear in selection interviews needs to be taken seriously, so that it may be determined whether this is something which training might temper or is so essential a part of the personality that it is unlikely to yield to any form of educational influence.

ii

We shall next consider selection from the candidates' side, noticing first the reasons which lead them to apply for admission. At the time of selection candidates give some account of their reason for wanting to enter the Mental Health Course, either in a letter accompanying their application form or in an essay. The question of motives is also very likely to be discussed at selection interviews. To this information, drawn from records of the Course, we are able to add from our present study information about their motives from nearly eighty of the subjects, who marked from among a list[1] of statements those which applied to themselves. We must be prepared to find motives of which subjects were only half aware at the time of selection reported for the first time at the study interview, and those reported at the time of application evidently forgotten.

From the nature and history of psychiatric social work we might expect candidates' motives for application to be mixed. When, as occasionally happens, only one motive is given, this may represent singleness of purpose or simplicity of personality, but may equally stand for a certain uneasiness in being interviewed. Thus a subject who admitted to a fear of giving herself away marked only the quite non-committal motive of wanting to qualify for psychiatric social work. It may be significant that, of those who failed or withdrew from the Course, three out of the fifteen who completed the schedule of motives had only one motive to report. Yet, although in the distinction group none of the fifteen who completed the schedule gave only a single motive, two gave only two. Most subjects, however, gave a larger range of motives, as many as nine in certain cases; these included a candidate, notably reserved and inarticulate when interviewed, who was able to mark on the schedule

[1] See Appendix II, p. 254.

several motives of a kind which might understandably have been avoided as too deeply self-revealing.

It may be useful to give an example of how motives may be combined. This subject has proved herself unusually intelligent, balanced, responsible and honest in her judgment of herself. Her achievement in psychiatric social work has been outstanding. On the schedule she marked eight motives, underlining the wish for a year at the university and for study as being especially important to her, which is easily understandable since she had no opportunity to study for a university degree. She is among the four who admitted a wish to earn a higher salary, and among the many who sought in the Course more understanding of the problems which they were meeting in work in which they were engaged. It may be characteristic that she had hoped through the Course to learn more about the workings of her own mind, but had not thought of it as a source of help in personal difficulties. It may also be regarded as characteristic of her general objective attitude that she noted that others had thought her suitable for this profession, rather than that she herself was aware of a natural ability to understand and help.

A considerable number of subjects were able to admit to the belief that they had some natural ability for understanding and helping people and to the wish to help individuals undergoing mental suffering. This appears to conflict with a tendency among social workers, noted by Margaret Mead,[1] to apologize for 'a simple desire to help human beings', of which indeed we ourselves found some evidence. Three went as far as to add that they wished to be in a position to help to prevent the unhappiness which they themselves had experienced in childhood and its consequences in later life. It is worth noting how matters worked out in their case. One failed in the Course. One qualified, but her time as a student was unhappy and her work uneven; the care of a young family has prevented her from practising as a psychiatric social worker. The third now holds successfully a very responsible post, but between her uneasy start in training and her present achievement lies a personal analysis.

Motives such as a wish for a higher salary, improved status or a break in one's occupation might be regarded as 'precipitating causes' for a candidate's application, and are as a rule combined

[1] Mead, Margaret: *Male and Female, A Study of the Sexes in a Changing World*, Gollancz, 1949, p. 305.

with several others which are of longer standing. The motive of which she is the most conscious at this point may fade in importance as she learns at first hand what it is into which she has been drawn, and as obscure motives become more clearly recognized. It does not seem to follow that the apparently casual candidate, who has 'happened to hear about the Mental Health Course', will not find as deep a satisfaction in psychiatric social work and do as well in it as one whose application has seemed more informed and purposive.

Hardly less important than the motives for application, and of course not unconnected with them, are the attitudes shown by candidates towards their selection; these, if the candidate is selected, are liable to be carried over into the training itself and may affect her ability to make good use of it. Aware that we are over-simplifying, we would divide the subjects of our study into three groups in accordance with the way in which they approached selection. There were those who approached it defensively, those who were convinced in advance of their own suitability and were mainly concerned with pressing their claims to be admitted, and those who were prepared to submit themselves, without defences, to the judgment of the people who were responsible for selection.

It might be thought that the first group had come like the second with minds made up about their own suitability, since they were obviously acting in a way likely to prevent them from gaining any useful vocational knowledge from the selection process. With a few this may have been true, but others were so obviously uncertain of themselves that we must look elsewhere for the cause of their defensiveness. In one candidate it seemed to represent a general habit, adopted in the face of any situation that challenged her by a person who was used to making her own way in life. Perhaps one might call hers a fencer's attitude in a contest which she certainly enjoyed ('it was rather a joke'), even though she was seriously concerned about the issue. A belief that her background and upbringing set her apart from other candidates and would be regarded unfavourably by the interviewers brought one candidate to her selection determined to give herself away as little as possible. She felt, in looking back, that she had been able to 'throw dust in people's eyes' and had kept up her defences quite successfully. One of those who did not qualify described herself as 'bluffing' her way through selection and told of her relief when she found herself outside the door after her interview with the psychiatrist, 'with no awkward questions asked'. Some, like the two just mentioned, had a fairly clear idea of what they were defending. In other cases, we think, the reserved and cautious mood in which they approached selection may have been more in the nature of a general response to rumours about how selection for the Mental Health Course was conducted.

Perhaps we too easily regard it as natural for selectors and candidates to be ranged against each other in a battle of wits. There are candidates who will have been assured by someone whose judgment they respect that they are eminently suitable for psychiatric social work; for them the main problem is to make their way into a closely guarded training. For these it may not be a question of concealing themselves at selection so much as of displaying their wares and frankly exposing their conviction. We refer in a later chapter to the sense of vocation among social workers. In the candidates we are now considering those responsible for selection are faced with a task which calls for an unusual degree of wisdom. A sincere conviction of one's own suitability, which cannot be treated lightly, may be combined with a different element, a tendency to 'gate-crash', which the barriers surrounding the Mental Health Course are liable to call out in a certain kind of personality. Such a candidate is not to be rejected *ipso facto*, yet it has to be considered that the training for which she feels herself so well suited is one in which she must be ready to become personally involved, and to find herself changing as a result. To learning and experiencing freely the attitude of the 'gate-crashing' candidate offers formidable obstacles.

The element of immaturity in many of the defensive candidates, as well as in those who insist upon their own suitability, reveals itself when these are compared with those who approach selection as a process in which candidates and interviewers meet together to solve a vocational problem. The subject who described this attitude most explicitly remarked that she had come to realize from talking later with professional colleagues that she was 'not a normal interviewee'. To her rejection would not have seemed disastrous, whereas admission under false pretences, or if she had been really unsuitable, would. Here she was thinking of her own good just as much as the profession's. She had known little about psychiatric social work when she had applied and had submitted herself to the interviews without any defences; she had no urgent feeling that she must be a psychiatric social worker and would not have had any sense of failure if she had been rejected. What she was sure about was that, having gained through her previous training a certain amount of psychological knowledge, she could not be a good social worker of any kind without more psychological training. She had thought that she could ask those responsible for the Course to suggest what she might do if they turned her down.

Interviewers are not responsible, unless very indirectly, for the attitudes with which candidates approach selection but cannot, of course, escape responsibility for the way they deal with them. If, for example, a particular candidate's attitude was defensive, it would obviously point to inadequate interviewing should the interviewer not recognize this. In certain circumstances, however, it might be a sign of wisdom rather than inadequacy for the interviewer, having recognized them, to respect the candidate's defences. Much can be learned from the defensive behaviour itself and from that part of the personality which is not concealed.

We notice that some candidates who now remember themselves as on the defensive at selection interviews are described by their interviewers as 'rather inhibited and shy', or as having an expression and manner which suggested underlying discouragement and anxiety. It is probably not by chance that two of them, whose energy presumably went into keeping up their defences, are described as lacking in vitality. On the whole, as one would expect, the defensive candidates did themselves less than justice. Yet this does not always apply. Two candidates, who described to us later how they defended at their interviews serious personal problems of which they were fully aware, made an excellent impression on all their interviewers, who did not seem to recognize the defensive attitudes described. We do not know why the defensiveness went apparently unrecognized by all the interviewers concerned. Some inadequacy in interviewing suggests itself, yet it may also be that the candidates were less generally defensive than they now consider themselves to have been. What is most important is that the positive qualities and the essential soundness of the personalities of these two candidates were recognized without hesitation at selection, so that what proved to be the right decision was made.

In a selection procedure in which those who interview, whether psychiatrist or psychiatric social worker, are often concerned in the training and in any case represent the kind of people with whom candidates may later have to work, we should expect candidates' feeling about the profession to which they are seeking admission to be a good deal influenced by what they think of their interviewers. As far as we can judge from our study disappointingly few use their interviews deliberately to help form their own judgment about whether this is the work for which they are best fitted and which they would like to take up, though more or less conscious judgments are undoubtedly being made all the time. One candidate had arranged before she was formally interviewed to see something of the work of several people who were engaged in training; in a sense, as she suggested, she was really interviewing them in relation to the Course, to see whether the people engaged in this work were the kind of people she herself would like to be. Her impression was mixed, but resulted in her deciding to join their ranks. The judgment of a second was more severe. When she first came up for selection, she regarded herself as so badly interviewed that she withdrew her application, since she was not 'going to sit at the feet' of people like these. On looking back, she realizes that her attitude was affected by her general state of mind at the time, and it is satisfactory to report that she finally entered the training and was awarded a mark of distinction at the end of it. Even on her first application, as she admitted, her interview with the psychiatrist felt like 'the meeting of two people having a good look at each other'.

There are more criticisms of superficial or clumsy interviewing than of interviewing which was regarded as unwarrantably intrusive, though a few such criticisms do occur. Sometimes the criticism combines the two, as when a candidate, who felt that one of the psychiatric social workers who interviewed her was unnecessarily curious about her personal life, resented not so much the questions asked as the too obviously tactful way in which they were put ('there was too much beating about the bush'). To one subject the interviews seemed too subtle, so that she did not know where she was. 'I felt the care with which I was treated created rather than relieved anxiety about how I was doing.'

Criticisms by those interviewed of psychiatrists and non-psychiatrists were not essentially different. One describes as part of an unsatisfactory interview how the psychiatrist interviewer charged her with being 'fed-up' with the job she was in at the time. This term she rejects as a false description of the discontent, up to then only partly understood, which led her to seek a change of work and adds: 'What I needed was someone to stress the creative aspect of that discontent, namely that I had reached the point when I had both given to and taken from that job all I could, but that my past could be used creatively in the new training I sought. Had I not been accepted for the Course, that charge, unresolved, might have proved both discouraging and destructive.' This is an important comment. While some mention certain interviews as 'superficial', a few regarded the whole procedure in this way. One would have resented it if she had not been admitted because she would have felt that she had not been given a chance to show her quality. Some, on the other hand, regarded what were apparently the same kind of interviews in a different way. The method of one particular interviewer, for instance, was often described as 'social'. As used by some subjects the word certainly implied superficial. Yet others look back on their 'social' interviews as friendly encounters which they appreciated, while some were discerning enough to realize that they might be as adequately summed up at an interview of this nature as in one conducted more formally. A few indeed, in their early days of innocence, attributed to their interviewers as a body almost magical powers, or the possession, as one put it, of a 'psychological X-ray', which could operate whatever form the interview took.

It was evident that subjects often regarded their interviews as more than a bare means of selection. One when she applied was very uncertain of her own capacity. From childhood onwards she received a good deal of criticism which seemed to pull in different directions. She had come to feel her career a failure and had never learnt to criticize her own work or to appreciate what was good in it. A very critical report from a social agency where she had worked as a student had thrown her into 'a pretty bad state of despondency'. All her interviews for the Mental Health Course she described as 'sane and reassuring', but in one interview especially she found someone who seemed willing to accept her as she was. Her bad report and her third-class degree were discussed with her and she found that she could talk of them without feeling 'terribly ashamed'. The effect of the interview was carried over into the Course itself, where she did well and which she greatly enjoyed. Through it she was helped to reconcile 'those earlier contrary opinions of sides of my character and my intelligence and to realize that there was truth in diverse assessment and why this was'. Another subject reported a selection interview which had, at the time, the effect of release from tension, yet had come in her memory to be associated with frustration and regret, since the relationship established with her interviewer, which she greatly valued, remained during training to a great extent undeveloped.

The far-reaching effect of selection interviews was touched upon from various standpoints. Some subjects recalled their interviews as reassuring, quite apart from the possible issue in selection, but a few criticized the way in which a topic, which would obviously prove emotionally disturbing, such as a family history of mental instability, was raised and handled by a particular interviewer. Again one subject left an interview with the impression that she was regarded as having been ill prepared for the Course academically. As a result, between her acceptance and the beginning of training, she read every book on a preliminary reading list and entered the Course with the idea that, unless she 'read like mad', she would not make good.

None of the subjects suggested any other means of selection than those in use, but we ourselves raised the question of how they would have felt if psychological tests had formed part of the procedure when they applied for admission. It was only on intelligence tests that we obtained any expression of opinion, and here the views of the subjects depended largely upon whether they had already had experience of such tests and what this had been. Those who were convinced, when they entered the Course, that they were below standard intellectually thought that such tests would have been very disturbing to them; one declared that she would have withdrawn her application rather than face them.

Our study of accepted candidates suggests that most regarded the procedure of selection for the Mental Health Course as fair. We were not able to explore the views of rejected candidates ; from these it is likely that we should have gained a very different picture. But it may be asked whether the candidate's views about this need be considered. Is it not enough if a decision is reached which proves, in the event, to have been a wise one? We have in mind, for example, the student already mentioned who considered the whole selection process to which she was subjected to have been superficial, only justifiable if it was merely a form and the decision reached on the basis of reports from referees on her previous achievement. In fact the reports on the interviews suggest that these were not unfruitful and that much was learned about this candidate, who was recognized from the first as full of promise. In view of her critical attitude towards selection it is worth noting that her attitude towards training was also critical, though much of the criticism was turned upon herself. From the standpoint of the training staff she passed out into employment as someone whose achievement as a student, though hardly fulfilling the expectations held at selection, suggested that she might ultimately make some original contribution to her profession. At the time of our study, after twelve years of varied experience, this subject was given by her psychiatrist referee the highest assessment, and an exceptionally detailed report on her work described a person of more than usual ability. What is to be said of the selection of this candidate, which was undoubtedly justified in its result if we think only in terms of a competent member added to the profession, but which apparently left her dissatisfied, because she herself felt that no one had taken the trouble to discern her real quality? We have seen how the influence of selection interviews can extend into training and we must ask ourselves whether, if the interviewers had been able to win the confidence of this essentially reserved candidate, her career as a student would not have been more fruitful and have left her with a more satisfying memory.

We must not, of course, base too much upon a single instance. What we are really concerned with is the general question of whether it is essential that justice should 'not only be done but should manifestly and undoubtedly be seen to be done.' Earlier in this chapter we have suggested that it is desirable that the selection interview should be regarded, by both parties, as a co-operative attempt to solve a vocational problem. If this were so, the whole situation would be changed. Both parties to the interview would accept it as natural that personal qualities were being assessed and both would feel responsible for providing the best conditions for reaching a solution. The aims of the parties, of course, are not identical; the candidate will naturally be chiefly concerned with her own career and the interviewer with seeking to secure for the professional training those best able to use it and most likely to make a valuable contribution to the profession. But the aims of the two are complementary, and anything which ensures, side by side with increasing skill on the part of those who interview, an increasing sense of responsibility in those who submit themselves for selection, is very well worth cultivating. We pointed out earlier that candidates reach selection already influenced by various rumours which circulate about the nature of the Mental Health Course and how one is admitted to it. In unfavourable rumours the dissatisfied candidate, who has doubted the fairness of the selection procedure and has not been made to feel her own responsibility in it, is likely to play a considerable part.

iii

It might well be thought that we have been too much concerned up to now with the by-products of selection. Important as the influence of a selection interview may be on a candidate's later career, its first object is, after all, prediction. It is this aspect of selection to which we shall now turn. Where admission to training depends as largely upon personal qualities as it is known to do in the Mental Health Course, failure in selection, as we have suggested, is an especially serious matter. Those concerned with it are under a strong obligation to learn all they can from cases where selection seems to have gone wrong. We shall therefore examine a group of fourteen subjects who formed part of our study, nine of whom were failed at the end of training by the examining board, and five advised to withdraw before the examination, because it had become evident that they had embarked upon a training for which they were not suited. We consider this group again in a chapter devoted to the question of 'personal difficulties' and a certain amount of overlapping is inevitable. In what follows our guiding line will be the idea of prediction, and what the factors are which seem to affect its validity.

In all fourteen instances those responsible for selection might be regarded as having failed in prediction. Yet here it is necessary to discriminate. Representing the combined conclusions of the three interviewers by a three-point scale, we find that none of these candidates were rated A, seven were rated B, and two C. In three cases there was too marked a difference between the interviewers' opinions for any rating to be given, and in two, belonging to the earlier period of the Course, the scantiness of the records also precluded a rating. Two kinds of faulty selection are involved. In the one, all or most of those responsible were fully aware that the admission of the candidate entailed a considerable risk, but recognized certain possibilities which training might develop. In the other it would seem that the factors which led to failure were overlooked at selection, or seriously underestimated. Even here, in the reports of one of the interviewers at least, we can often see, retrospectively, a hint of some quality which contributed to failure;

in some cases this could hardly have been correctly interpreted before the candidate had been put to the test of training.

In those graded C, a large element of risk was recognized, as in the case of a candidate of sterling qualities, but of an apparently restricted outlook. There was considerable doubt whether she was capable of making the amount of adjustment which the Course would inevitably demand of her, but the interviewer with whom she talked most freely considered that she was now in a stage of rapid intellectual development, and was 'likely to meet frankly any clash between beliefs and further learning'.

At first sight it would seem that all those rated B at selection represented a real failure in prediction. Yet a B rating might also cover a clear recognition of risk, in the case of candidates who showed certain favourable qualities to a high degree. Moreover, in estimating risk, allowance is sometimes made for unusually adverse circumstances in the candidate's past. In one case, where risk was known to be high, it was recognized that the candidate, enterprising and full of eagerness but, as one interviewer described her, still 'untempered', had suffered severely from lack of stability in her early environment and might, if rightly handled, find her balance in the process of training. Looking back at the records, it is hard to see the risk as legitimate, yet this decision was based on no less than six individual interviews.

In a few cases selection seems to have been influenced by what might be termed an extraneous reason, as when a candidate proposed to return to a post for which the training offered by the Mental Health Course was held to be very desirable, or possessed qualifications which would fit her to hold some important position, if she could add to them that of the Course. Such extraneous reasons, while they may be allowed to turn the scale when personal claims to admission are moderately strong, need, in our experience, to be very carefully scrutinized.

We notice that half the present group of subjects were trained during the period of the war.[1] This is certainly striking. There can be no doubt that during these years selection and training were rendered more difficult by war conditions and that individual students were subjected to special strain. In some cases the war

[1] In our study of those who failed to qualify, we covered sessions 1931–32 to 1946–47. Of the British women who entered during this period somewhat over 7 per cent did not qualify; of these some withdrew for reasons other than unsuitability.

impinged particularly closely upon a student's personal life. One of those who failed still feels strongly that she should have been encouraged to suspend her training for this reason; another, who found herself becoming increasingly preoccupied with personal anxieties related to war conditions, did in fact withdraw from the Course, to return some years later and complete it successfully. Yet the particular circumstances of the war years can never be more than a partial explanation and it is probably wiser not to isolate this group of 'failures' from the rest.

Considering candidates' formal qualifications, we take first that of age. Preference in awarding scholarships for the Course was given to candidates from the age of twenty-five to thirty-five because experience suggested that fewer casualties were to be expected within this span. Among the fourteen subjects of our present group the ages of nine lie within these years, none below and five above. The proportion of older students is certainly higher in this group than that found among subjects as a whole. Nevertheless, while we would not minimize the importance of age on admission and realize that older students are likely to use the training somewhat differently from the students of the lower and middle age groups, our experience suggests that in selection the mere fact of chronological age can be misleading. We are reminded of a candidate, not included in our study, who was admitted to training in her middle fifties. Doubts about her admission were felt, not only because of her age but because her qualifications did not conform closely with those laid down for the Course. Yet she not only completed her training successfully, but has at the time of writing given fifteen years of unbroken and valuable service as a psychiatric social worker.

There was no university degree among the fourteen candidates, but all except two held social science certificates.[1] Experience before admission to the Course was so varied among these candidates that it is difficult to relate it in any significant way to the fact of failure. One general observation, however, is perhaps worth recording. We did not find in the careers of any of these subjects a continuous sequence from school to social science training and so on to a salaried post in social work, followed in due course by an application for admission to the Mental Health Course—a pattern

[1] Of the seventy-one subjects who qualified, eight had a degree only, twenty had a degree and social science certificate, and thirty-six a social science certificate only. Seven had neither qualification.

which is not uncommon in the careers of those who qualified. We are anxious that this fact should not be misinterpreted. The variety of the past careers of those who enter the Course is something which we value highly, both for the training and for the profession. For individuals too a variety of experience, especially such as brings first-hand knowledge of conditions far removed from those in which they have grown up, can form an admirable basis for the later specialized training. Where the social science training and experience in social work come in the whole sequence is often a matter of circumstances not altogether within the individual's control; we do not believe that any one sequence is necessarily the best. There are psychiatric social workers doing work of special value, whose careers before the Course were no more orthodox than those which might be thought of as characteristic of our present group. This fact offers a particular challenge to skill in prediction. At certain points in many careers it would be hard to judge how far the tentative, zigzagging course which it has presented hitherto points to fundamental instability and dissatisfaction, is mainly the effect of special circumstances, or is an indication of unusual initiative and persistence in following a partly unconscious purpose, which might perhaps be realized in psychiatric social work.

We shall give from this group a single example of the interplay of factors which has to be taken into account when a decision about admission to the Course is made. From one referee we learn that this subject came up from school to enter the social science course of one of the universities with a reputation for cleverness, which did not 'materialize as intelligence'. She had gained her social science certificate but failed to qualify in the special form of social work for which she had entered, even with an extended period of training. The reports of those who supervised her work during this time show surprising differences of opinion, but when they are adverse the traits they mention, while serious in any profession, are those likely to be particularly damaging in psychiatric social work. One of the referees, who was in a position to compare this training with the Mental Health Course, could not believe that this subject would succeed in the very specialized training for which she was now applying, unless in the meantime she had overcome the difficulties of personality which had led to previous failure. This of course was the crux of the matter, and it must be pointed out, in defence of her selection for the Mental Health

Course, that a period of very successful work with children, carried on in most difficult conditions, had given reason to hope that a change had really taken place. Another referee, well qualified to judge, thought highly of her work here and regarded her as intellectually quite up to the standard of the Course and likely to make considerable progress during the year. Interviewers were aware of the candidate's immaturity, but were ready to believe that, while she had been slow to develop, she was now developing fast. Her lack of success in the earlier training might have reflected a phase of personal difficulties from which she was now emerging; these might have been accentuated by the fact of training for a particular profession for which she was essentially unsuitable.

Here then was a candidate about whom there was no lack of information at the time of her application, and who was interviewed by four people, including two psychiatrists. While it was realized that the Mental Health Course was only an approximation to the course she was needing, in which the emphasis would have been on skill in direct work with children, yet the comment that she 'should do quite a good job of work as a psychiatric social worker' seems to be a fair summary of all the interviewers' conclusions. The failure in training which followed involved both academic and practical work, and the wisdom of the examining board's decision can hardly be questioned. In view of the excellent reports on this candidate's work just before admission, we assume that the falseness of her position in this particular kind of training caused her to do herself less than justice. She now holds a very responsible job in social work along the lines of her special interests, and in a two-years period had already been promoted. In answer to our questionnaire she replied that she was satisfied that her present work was, on the whole, the kind for which she was best suited.

With those who failed to qualify we can only say that hopes formed at selection were not fulfilled; the decision then made excluded them from the test of employment, where they might have made good. With those who qualified the question of prediction is more complex. For nearly all the qualified subjects of our study we have some knowledge of their careers after training, but the amount varies widely. We shall confine ourselves here to a group of forty-two qualified subjects about whom we obtained an assessment on their achievement as psychiatric social workers from a psychiatrist referee.[1] In the following table certain facts about the relations between their assessment in selection, training and employment are set out. We have disregarded here the assessment of second referees, who were not psychiatrists, though their answers to our questions are drawn upon in other contexts.

ASSESSMENTS COMPARED

	i *Training with Selection*	ii *Employment with Training*	iii *Employment with Selection*
Higher			
(considerably)	1	2	1
(somewhat)	20	9	23
Similar	16	25	16
Lower			
(considerably)	0	0	0
(somewhat)	5	6	2
	42	42	42

Passing from a group of subjects who, to judge by their failure to qualify, were overestimated at selection, we are struck in the table given above by the evidence of a contrary tendency. This impression is reinforced by the records of those subjects for whom we did not obtain a psychiatrist's assessment on their work, and who are therefore not represented in the table; ten out of twenty-six[2] of these appeared better in training than in selection, and only one less good, and we have no reason to think that the assessment of employment, had we obtained one, would not, in the majority of cases, have been at least as high as for training. The upward trend in the forty-two covered by column ii supports this. This tendency to underestimate calls for careful attention, since it involves the possibility that some of the candidates rejected at selection might have made good in training. A study of what happened to rejected candidates would be instructive, if it were sufficiently detailed and penetrating; the fact that a rejected candidate did well in some other type of work would not decide whether rejection for the Mental Health Course had been justified.

[1] There were various reasons for not obtaining this assessment for the remaining twenty-nine qualified subjects, none of which seems to affect the inferences to be drawn from the table.

[2] For three of the twenty-nine referred to above, selection records were too scanty to allow of a rating.

Among the subjects of our study who qualified, there are sixteen from the same span of years as those who failed, who were awarded a mark of distinction. What this represented was understood rather than formulated: in some cases there was an unusually balanced achievement at a high level; in others, while work was of a good general standard, a somewhat less well balanced achievement was compensated for by evidence of originality and by the promise of an outstanding contribution to psychiatric social work in the future. It is worth considering whether the qualities of this group were conspicuous enough at selection to save those responsible from their besetting tendency. In fact the 'distinction' of these subjects did not prevent some from being underestimated. While the A qualities of eight were recognized at selection, seven were assessed as B.[1] Such cases should be particularly instructive. In the distinction group are two whom we considered earlier in this chapter who, on their own showing, were on the defensive at their interview and as a result did not reveal their positive qualities. One of them who, as a student, was reported to have shown an independent mind, and sensitiveness and imagination in dealing with people and as being a fearless and tolerant critic of her own work, impressed one of her interviewers as a 'B worker with enough understanding for good case-work, but without much originality or drive', and as showing the limitations of a person of rather one-sided experience. The other, whose defensive attitude seems to have been shown to one only of her interviewers, was characterized in general by a kind of friendly shyness. Her tendency to do herself less than justice was noted during training by her tutor, who was afraid that a cynical attitude, which she herself recognized as protective, might tell against her in seeking employment. This does not in fact appear to have happened, and her psychiatrist referee ascribes to her 'an original and stimulating outlook'. This was certainly not appreciated until the stage of training.

A third subject from the distinction group presented an unusually difficult problem of selection. Well qualified academically and practically, she received high praise from her referees, yet one of them, who was fully acquainted with the demands of the training, would not have selected her as an ideal candidate; she suggested nevertheless that she had qualities upon which the Course might build. She added, as a hint to interviewers, that

[1] The selection records of the sixteenth were inadequate.

considerable force of character lay hidden behind a rather unimpressive façade. This façade, in the form of a somewhat stilted manner, gave the interviewers some trouble; one, for instance, saw it as a 'matter of general style' rather than as an implication of nervous tension, but to another the tension was very apparent. While in personal relations she gave the impression of being rather too precise and detached, it was also noted that each move in her career had been towards more direct contact with individuals. About her intelligence, good judgment and sensitive understanding of other people there seems to have been no doubt at all. The opinion of the psychiatrist who interviewed her was, however, quite definite; he regarded her as needing analysis or some personal readjustment to render her suitable for psychiatric social work. In spite of this the Selection Committee took the risk of admitting her and her subsequent career, after a singularly successful period of training, is of interest. Her psychiatrist referee, writing of her as he knew her several years before the time of our study, referred appreciatively to most aspects of her work and in the highest terms to her capacity for research. An unevenness in more intensive case-work suggested, however, the presence of personal problems such as the advice of the psychiatrist who interviewed her would seem to have foreshadowed. The referee's further comment is worth quoting, in view of what had actually happened at selection. After describing her intelligence as so high 'that even with a bad training she would have been a good and valuable collaborator', he added: 'Her emotional troubles were of such a nature that I do not think any selection could have detected them before (the candidate) had been put under the strain of psychiatric work.' This career, which includes subsequent posts of a specially exacting and responsible kind, is one which can only be adequately assessed after the lapse of a considerable period of time.

Overestimation at selection we have considered already in the case of those who failed to qualify. Among those who qualified this tendency can also be illustrated, but the proportion of those to whom it applies is exceedingly small. Among the forty-two subjects for whom we have a psychiatrist's assessment of their work, only one shows a high assessment at selection followed by a lower assessment both in training and practice. It should be useful to study her record.

This candidate's previous career conformed with the qualifications laid down for the Course and she held a university degree.

Her referees, who included a psychiatric social worker, all recommended her as suitable for admission. There appears to have been complete unanimity among her interviewers about her suitability as a scholarship candidate; we must therefore assume that the interviewer who thought her manner slightly superficial and noted her anxiety to make a good impression did not regard these as serious warnings of difficulties to come. Beyond a reference to her interest in psychology, there is little in the records to indicate why this candidate was thought of as fitted for psychiatric social work; the stress is laid rather on her social qualities, such as good appearance, ability to talk intelligently on matters of general interest and the fact that she had behind her a favourable social and educational background. During training good qualities were noted in all aspects of her work, but also certain difficulties which prevented her from using her considerable abilities freely. One supervisor reported a rigidity of mind which caused her to overlook the more subtle problems in case-work; another mentioned that she showed tension in relations with her fellow workers, and difficulty in accepting any criticism of her work. Her tutor reported well of her academic work and noted that she seemed modest about her achievements, adding that she sometimes gave the impression that her critical judgments were too facile. With regard to employment her psychiatrist referee reported excellent abilities and good psychological insight. Difficulties of personality, however, had seriously affected her relationship with other members of the staff, causing at times a deterioration of her work as a whole. 'If she had more insight into her own reactions (i.e., if she were analysed), she would be a first-class psychiatric social worker.' We think that it must be admitted that the interviewing of this candidate was less than adequate. Greater understanding at selection might have led to an earlier appreciation of her difficulties in the training period and so to a greater possibility of helping her to solve them. Yet, as her referee implied, it is doubtful whether they were amenable to educational methods.

When overestimation occurs in other instances, either training shows a lower assessment than selection with a return to the selection level in employment, or, after a training which seems to confirm the judgment made at selection, the level drops when it comes to employment. We shall consider some of these cases later.

The best evidence of good selection is obviously an assessment which corresponds with that for both the other phases. This is not shown on our table, but exists in fact in the case of nine out of the forty-two subjects, seven of whom received the highest and two the middle rating. When we think of the seven as individuals, an interesting point emerges. It would not be unreasonable to assume that these subjects, who made such a consistently good impression at all three phases, would be characterized by the evenness of their temperaments and the uneventfulness of their careers. This is by no means how we think of them. It is true that their high assessment in training and employment points to an essential soundness of personality or at least to a sense of professional responsibility, which prevented such personal difficulties as they carried from making themselves felt beyond reasonable limits in their work. But these are not subjects whom we remember as imperturbable students and in the case of some of them we know that the period of training was marked by more, rather than less, than the usual degree of stress. This is not irrelevant to the question of the kind of stability to be demanded of a candidate for training in the Mental Health Course, which we discuss in Chapter X.

In considering the use of the interview in selection, we have had in mind chiefly the single interview. In the selection procedure, however, this never stood alone, but formed part of a succession of individual interviews, normally by three persons. No plan was imposed on the interviewers, and this freedom, provided that the interviewers are clear about their common purpose, seems to us valuable. Even in the absence of full records, which has made our task more difficult, it is clear that the separate interviewers not only had their own ideas of what a selection interview should be, but often called out, through their different personalities, very different responses from the candidates, so that when they came to formulate a judgment each, to some extent, based his or her conclusions on different material. One interviewer will tend to find candidates withdrawn and enigmatic, while with another the same candidates have clearly opened out with a normal degree of confidence and frankness. It is also possible to detect in some cases differences in the value attached by individual interviewers to the attitudes which candidates display. With one interviewer any sign of self-assertion tends to be faintly suspect, while with another it is taken to represent, if not too pronounced, a good basis for training. One interviewer, again, is apt to be impressed in advance by wide cultural and educational advantages, while another will be biased in favour of experiences which have called for initiative and endurance. Our study provided us with two examples of a difference of appreciation among interviewers of the value of the latter kind of experience; one of these candidates was failed by the examining board, while the other, after making excellent use of training, has shown outstanding ability in her profession.

Ideally, in arranging for a candidate a series of interviews, the known characteristics of interviewers should be taken into account. This is not always practicable but, even without it, we have no doubt that there is value in a candidate being seen by more than one interviewer, for which a succession of interviews by a single person could hardly compensate. All experienced interviewers for the Mental Health Course would probably agree that there is apt to develop in their minds a conception of a psychiatric social worker, against which they tend to measure those they interview. This, if it remains unexamined and unchecked, may easily become stereotyped along the lines of their own idiosyncrasies. This tendency is to a great extent rendered innocuous when reports of the several interviewers are pooled through a selection committee, where the individual stereotypes may be broken down.

We made a special point in our study of noticing what kind of contribution the psychiatrist appeared to be making at a time when his position was not, as it was later to become, that of a consultant in cases of possible psychiatric difficulty, but of a member of a team of interviewers, concerned like the rest with the problems of selection as a whole. This position could be justified on several grounds. One might think of the psychiatrist as likely, because of his training and experience, to be an especially skilled interviewer, or consider that his advice was obviously desirable in selecting for a profession which is often thought of as attracting unstable people and as stirring up emotional problems; or again, since psychiatrists and psychiatric social workers are associated during and after training, it might be thought appropriate to introduce the psychiatrist at the selection stage. It should be noted that the psychiatrists who interviewed for selection had, in some cases, taken part in the training and in all had experience of working with those who had been trained. As far as we could judge from our study, candidates accepted the interview with a psychiatrist as quite natural, being sometimes appreciative, sometimes critical, as they were of other interviews. In almost every case where we know that the interview was especially thorough and psychiatric in nature the candidate seems to have understood it in terms of the work she hoped to take up. Some psychiatrists evidently conducted their interviews very much as did their lay colleagues, while the interviews of others, to judge from the reports, approximated to a psychiatric examination. This of course will have depended partly, but not wholly, upon whether or not they had been asked to give an opinion as an expert as well as a member of the interviewing team. A few illustrations should bring out more clearly the part in selection which a psychiatrist may play.

We have already mentioned a psychiatrist interviewer who regarded a candidate as unsuitable for training without psychotherapeutic help. In this case a risk was taken and the candidate admitted, against the psychiatrist's advice since she did not first receive the help he recommended. On the wisdom of the decision from the standpoint of the candidate's development and peace of mind we can give no judgment; from the standpoint of the profession we can only regard the decision as amply justified.

In the second instance the candidate's later career fully bore out the psychiatrist's report. He described her as 'intelligent though not original', 'most well-balanced, entirely practical, without much subtlety or after-thought, self-analysis or more than superficial analysis of others. Very good indeed for anything less than refined characterological research.' This might be regarded as a psychiatric assessment, but it is to be noted that essentially the same conclusions were reached by the other two interviewers, and indeed it would have been hard to avoid them.

The third candidate had passed through personal experiences which might, it was thought, have made it undesirable for her to take the Mental Health Course. Interviews with two psychiatrists were arranged; one of these concluded that she was well adjusted to work with cases of mental disorder, in spite of experiences which had brought her into contact with it in a painfully intimate way; the other, even though he recognized that her interest was based upon personal circumstances, did not believe that she would be unduly disturbed by the Course—judgments which were fully borne out by her record during and after training.

About the suitability of a fourth candidate there was general hesitation. The psychiatrist, after careful interviewing, reported that, if an emotional change could be effected, she might prove capable of first-class work, but that it was doubtful whether she would change appreciably. It was a 'toss-up' dependent upon her capacity to learn. It was decided to take the risk of admitting her, but her training was a troubled one, ending in failure. Looking back, one may doubt whether the necessary emotional change could, in any case, have been effected in a single year of training or through educational means alone. Here, as always, problems of selection and problems of training hang together. A combination of circumstances which did not happen, a greater capacity on the part of some member of the training staff to establish a relationship within which learning could have taken place, and the 'toss-up' might have gone the other way.

Three of the psychiatrists who contributed to our study stressed the extreme difficulty of selection interviewing. One pointed out that comparatively few psychiatrists could assess at a single interview. 'Very quick insight is needed into character and motives, conscious and particularly less conscious.' Two felt that a personal psychiatric examination was really what was needed—('It is so easy to be deceived by a good *persona*')—yet both hesitated to impose this upon a candidate. It seems possible that the psychiatrists' special experience and training may have made it more rather than less difficult for some to interview for the purpose of selection. Unfortunately our study did not yield any decisive answer to the question which we had specially in mind—whether, because of such experience and training, psychiatrists could be shown to have made an indispensable contribution to selection where no specifically psychiatric problems seemed to be involved. The most that can be said is that, judged by our comparatively small study, psychiatrists do not seem to us to have contributed a special kind of judgment to the work of the interviewing team or recognized potential failures more accurately than interviewers without a psychiatrist's training. There may, however, be other good reasons for a psychiatrist to share in the general task of selection.

Behind the individual interviews we have always assumed the presence of a selection committee, which does not itself see the candidates but, weighing the reports of the separate interviewers together with information about the candidates' past careers, reaches the final decision about admission. Why, it might be asked, should not the procedure be simplified by cutting out the part of the individual interviewers and substituting an interview by the committee, which would then reach its decision on the basis of the members' immediate impression of the candidate? There are two main questions involved: whether the interviews with individuals could be abolished without serious loss and whether there is a positive value in a candidate's appearing before such a committee.

Part of the answer to the first question has been provided by the earlier sections of this chapter. It should have become clear that, although the nature and degree of intimacy of what is discussed at individual interviews will vary widely from one to another, candidates will often at a private interview raise problems or give information which they would be unlikely to entrust to a committee, however informal and sympathetic. In many cases such material has proved important in reaching a decision on selection, but besides this, if interviewer and candidate are able to establish a good relation, this can prove of positive value to the candidate in thinking through her vocational problems, where personal and professional issues are often intermixed.

It is obviously reasonable that as part of the process of selecting candidates to train for a profession in which the personal interview plays so important a part, she should herself be assessed in this same situation, however different her rôle in it may be from the one she would have to sustain after admission. Yet the functions of psychiatric social workers are not confined to personal interviewing. A candidate's ability to enter into relations with groups, and to get her case across to them, would presumably be more adequately assessed at a committee interview than through contact with single individuals. The use of a committee interview in addition to individual interviews has therefore much to commend it. But it would not then simplify selection procedure and, from the candidate's point of view, would greatly add to the trials of what has often been criticized as an unnecessarily elaborate ordeal. One psychiatrist referee writes: 'I would advocate the present personal interview plus an interview by the whole committee—at least in cases where there is any doubt at all either way', and adds: 'On looking back over the few failures in training I have come across personally, I am sure they would have been spotted by an interview of this sort; or at least come under suspicion.' This may well be, yet it has been comparatively rare in the Mental Health Course for students who failed to have passed through the selection interviews without having aroused a suspicion with regard to their suitability.

In selection such as we are considering it is important to remind ourselves what it is that is being assessed. It is certainly not a bundle of personality traits. One of the strongest impressions left by our present study is that when prediction is faulty in any direction, it has not been mainly a matter of blindness at selection to certain single traits which have revealed themselves as undesirable at a later stage, but rather of a failure to realize what a personality, scrutinized at a given time under artificial conditions, is likely to become when subjected to the partly foreseeable and partly quite unforeseeable influences and stresses of training, followed by the even less predictable experiences of a career in a still very fluid profession. For this kind of prediction the metaphor of a 'psychological X-ray', which one subject attributed to her selectors, is much too static.

It may well be that the kind of imaginative foresight required for the final decision in selection would be more easily achieved by a committee, on a first hand impression of the candidate than on reports alone. This seems likely on the face of it. It is easy to discount a tentative suggestion of risk or promise in the report of an interviewer, less easy to undervalue it when it reaches one through direct contact. The increased attention given in recent years to the way people work together in groups should help to throw light on this. In the meantime we are convinced, on the basis of our study and of our general experience, that the method of interviewing individually by at least two persons who are familiar both with the training and the nature of the work for which it prepares has been shown to be reasonably successful. Other methods should be regarded as subsidiary and be planned with careful consideration of their effect upon the central process.

It is sometimes suggested that, in the present state of knowledge, only 'negative selection' is possible and that all candidates with the formal qualifications required, and not obviously unfitted on the grounds of personality, should be freely admitted for probationary training. In this case, it is assumed, a less elaborate process of selection would meet the case. This is debatable. We hope that the whole trend of this chapter will have dispelled any idea that 'negative selection' is likely to be a simple matter. Moreover, the difficulties involved, when it comes to training, in having admitted a large number of students with the expectation that a considerable number will prove personally unsuitable should be-become obvious from the discussion of training which follows. This method in any case would hardly make for economy.

There is an alternative proposal which goes some way to meet this difficulty and has a bearing also upon the present shortage of trained psychiatric social workers.[1] This is the proposal that prospective students should try themselves out in the field of psychiatric social work under adequate supervision, before being actually admitted to training. The question of supervision is of course crucial, if only because on its nature will depend, to a great extent, the spirit, receptive or otherwise, in which an individual will later approach formal training. A psychiatrist referee who outlines such a plan writes: 'During such a practical traineeship of, say, six months, it would be easy to eliminate unsuitable persons and to get the opinion of a number of independent observers on the candidate. To start with practical work would also take away the peculiar academic flavour and conceit of which some psychiatric social workers never rid themselves entirely.'[2] There is clearly much to be said for 'trainee' schemes, but they do not, as it seems to us, obviate the need to select candidates on the grounds of personality for the 'traineeship' itself. Trainees, like psychiatric social workers in training and after, will be involved in responsible work with individuals under the particular stress which attaches to mental illness and, in the nature of the case, are likely to be under less close supervision than students under formal training. The duty to safeguard the welfare of those at whose expense professional learning takes place needs to be frequently brought to mind. We shall return to this in the chapter on training which follows.

[1] Cf. the trainee scheme recommended by the Mackintosh Report (par. 128–33) to meet the shortage in psychiatric social workers. Such a scheme is at present in force, on a small scale, in mental hospitals, organized by the Association of Psychiatric Social Workers. Selection for this, in which a candidate is interviewed by one person and also by three together, does not appear to be less thorough than that for the Mental Health Course itself.

[2] We consider this line of criticism in Chapter IX.

CHAPTER V

TRAINING

i

We have already given a short account of the form and content of the London Mental Health Course as we have known it. A course of training must always seem very different to those responsible for training and to the students undergoing it. We therefore particularly welcome the memories of their training and their views about it contributed by subjects of our study, and have used these freely throughout this chapter.

We have tried to show how the Mental Health Course arose out of a convergence of different needs and interests, and how easily the curriculum might have become confused. In so far as this has been avoided it would seem to be because the Course has been planned as a whole and has been held together, not only by a committee representing the varied interests involved, formed for the special purpose of advising the London School of Economics about the Course, but also by the frequent informal consultation of those taking a direct part in theoretical and practical training.

We shall consider first what students thought about the Course as a whole. Many understandably considered it too short and a few would have liked more time for reading. Most, however, at least in retrospect, did not think that they felt unduly rushed; some even felt a sense of leisure after the heavy posts from which they had just come. Many spoke of the training as something they had enjoyed in a most positive way[1]; several of these mentioned too that they had for this reason accepted it rather naïvely and uncritically. One intelligent and quite experienced subject, who had enjoyed

[1] Of the ninety-three subjects there were seven qualified and seven unqualified who did not take part in the study. Their views might have added significantly to the criticism which we received on training.

its 'newness', described herself as having 'mopped it up'. A less experienced but equally intelligent subject wrote that she had accepted the Course as it stood 'in the simple belief that it was offered because it was known to be appropriate experience and training'. This tendency to accept the planning of the Course as a whole is notable in a body of students who could be healthily critical of detail.

We asked some of the subjects how far the Course had seemed to them well integrated and received a variety of replies. Some had evidently given little thought to the relation of parts to whole. As one would expect, what the Course meant to each seemed to be determined by what she herself brought to it. One subject, with an unusually critical mind, found it stimulating to meet with such a variety of opinion within the training and would have liked the lectures to have been more provocative. Another was 'so worried about reaching an adequate standard on the *academic* side' that she had 'little time to be concerned about other aspects'.

It is important to remember that the Course came to different students at different points in their careers. We take four examples from our study. The first subject entered the training in her early thirties. Her degree course had been interrupted through illness; later she had been engaged for some years in research as remote as could well be conceived from the work to which she was now attracted. She was admitted after completing a specially arranged training in social work. The second, in her late thirties, had been engaged for many years in clerical work before breaking off to undertake a university course in social science, which she had just successfully completed when she was admitted to the Mental Health Course. The third was admitted in her early twenties; the Course followed hard upon a diploma in social science, which had been preceded immediately by a degree at the same university. The fourth, who entered in her middle twenties, held a university degree and a social science certificate of the same university. A period of social work separated this period of training from the Mental Health Course. Such bare outlines do scant justice to the actual variety in the past careers of students entering the Course. A study which related a student's past career with her experience both during training and after qualification might prove well worth making; it would be interesting to know, for instance, about the value of an interval between school or degree course and a course in social science, filled with experiences of a quite different kind from those in which the individual will become involved as a professional social worker.[1] It is important to know such things in planning for any modification in training for social work, especially if an extension of the period of training is contemplated.

In an earlier chapter we imagined a social worker, faced in her job with the problems of personality and relationship which baffled her understanding, awaiting enlightenment from some field beyond her own. A number of these entered the Mental Health Course, and, although some finally decided to work with the mentally ill or maladjusted, some kept to their original intention of returning to a form of social work not specifically psychiatric. From the title of the Course they would have been justified in expecting to find in it an emphasis upon positive mental health and the prevention of mental illness, rather than its treatment. It is worth while considering what in fact they would have met there.

A first examination of the contents of the Mental Health Course as we knew it would suggest that the emphasis in this training was, in fact, strongly upon mental ill-health. Teaching in clinical psychiatry and mental deficiency, together with continuous case-work on clinical material, might seem to outweigh such courses as those on the development of personality, psychological measurement and other problems of normal psychology, and on the historical background of the mental health services, thus giving the Course a definite tilt towards pathology. About this situation there are several comments to make. First, much knowledge in the field of normal psychology has its origin in the exploration of abnormal conditions, and this may be in some respects the most profitable sequence of study for each individual student. There is also, of course, a very practical reason for the Course's emphasis upon mental disorder. The training has to provide in the first place for social workers who will take up posts in association with clinical psychiatry, and for this purpose more and not less than the present amount of teaching in psychiatry is desirable.[2]

It is easy to make here too clear-cut a distinction. It would be generally agreed that the student who expects to work after qualification as a psychiatric social worker needs more than a formal knowledge of the elements of psychiatry. In the short time the

[1] Cf. pp. 75–6.

[2] The Mackintosh Report (par. 124 (iv)) suggests that 'more attention should be given in the mental health course to abnormal mental states'.

Course allows her she has also to lay the foundations of a knowledge of what mental illness means to the patient himself in his social relations and of what it means also in terms of disturbance and suffering to those in his environment. Such knowledge should be built upon the widest and most varied possible experience of people who come within the range of normality. In this the needs of the two groups of students, those intending to specialize and those returning to their former type of work, coincide. This is one of the reasons why a candidate's previous opportunities for such experience and her capacity to respond to it are given such careful consideration at selection. It cannot be left to the Course to provide this,[1] although, because the psychiatric social worker is largely concerned with members of the patient's environment she is adding all the time, in her training and later experience, to her range of knowledge of personality and behaviour in persons accepted as mentally healthy. This enlarging of experience of the 'normal' and the relating of it to the new insight which the Course should provide run concurrently with the study of pathological conditions. The behaviour of those not mentally ill may form a considerable part of the material studied by students with their supervisors, who, with the tutors, carry much of the responsibility for ensuring that students leave the Course with a concern for positive mental health.

A one year's course as wide in scope as the Mental Health Course lays itself open to the charge of being superficial. There is, of course, a sense in which this is true. Students of such a course cannot go deeply into any of the various subjects to which they are introduced by experts. Their study of psychiatry, for instance, is limited from the beginning, as many have felt keenly, by the lack of a medical training. In the same way the foundation of their study of psychology will not be that of a psychologist. Yet we believe that it is possible for the specialist to present his subject to someone who does not expect to make it his own without encouraging the latter to think superficially. On the contrary, the non-specialist student can be stimulated by the expert to the point where he begins to make his own application of the new subject, in

[1] Several subjects urged that experience with normal children should be included in the Course, if only to remind the student, while studying pathological conditions, of the variety of behaviour which lies within the range of normal development. A similar plea is made in an article, 'Practice versus Theory', by the Parents' Group of the Association of Psychiatric Social Workers: *British Journal of Psychiatric Social Work*, 5, 1951, p. 25.

that field of knowledge in which his feet are already firmly planted.

We do not claim that this difficult process has ever been achieved by the Course in a way which meets the needs of all, or even of most, of its students. There is a real danger that those who cannot tolerate the inevitable limitations of their knowledge of psychiatry, a field towards which they are likely to be drawn by a specially deep attraction, will react in various ways unfortunate for their future profession. While some, overwhelmed by their ignorance, will become discouraged and fail to develop confidence enough to offer a contribution of their own, others will make claims which, as it appears to others, they can neither formulate nor substantiate. It would seem to be some such confused claims which puzzled one of the psychiatrist referees, who found in the statements of some psychiatric social workers, though not of those with whom he worked, 'a mystical belief in themselves' and a tendency to refer always to the psychiatrist's limitations in the social field without apparently recognizing any limitations of their own. We do know, however, that neither of these attitudes is the inevitable result of the Mental Health Course, and that by those for whom, as one student put it, the Course has 'set the ball rolling', the 'superficial' knowledge acquired can be increasingly incorporated and may result in a kind of understanding and skill which has its own hall-mark.

ii

In this section we shall be concerned with ways of learning,[1] especially with learning through that personal interchange between staff and students which characterizes the Mental Health Course. Lectures, classes, discussion groups and clinical conferences, which take place concurrently, will be less often mentioned, but it is important to remember that the more individual forms of learning occur against this background.

The Course as we knew it covered about ten months. Qualification involves the satisfying of a Board of Examiners in written papers, and the attaining of a certain standard of academic work throughout the year. Practical training is no less involved and students have to adjust themselves to two training centres, differing

[1] Much of what is discussed in this chapter applies to the London Mental Health Course at all periods and, *mutatis mutandis*, to the Edinburgh and Manchester courses. We would again emphasize, however, that any description of procedure applies only to the London course as we knew it, even when, as is sometimes convenient, we use the present tense.

considerably in organization and outlook and in the part played there by the psychiatric social worker. Each student, even when her bent is markedly towards work with children or work with adults, has to reach a certain standard of competence in both, and there is a careful stock-taking, in which the student shares, when she passes from one centre to another; reports on both types of practical work form part of the information upon which the Board reaches its decision.

This is the structure within which each student works, where the general, inexorable time factor has to be accepted and the discipline which it imposes turned to account. But the variety existing among students of this Course has never allowed that other time factor to be forgotten, the characteristic tempo of the individual student. Many people take part in the training—lecturers in various subjects, psychiatrists, psychologists and others at the centre of academic teaching and, directly or indirectly, a variety of people at both centres of practical training. What we shall now chiefly consider is the work of those members of the training staff who have direct, individual and continuous contact with students—the tutors and supervisors. It is with these that the responsibility for this second time factor chiefly lies.

Throughout the greater part of the training academic and practical work run side by side. This can have a very different significance for different students. Our evidence suggests that while it is stimulating to some, for others it can be disrupting; we refer elsewhere to a subject who declared that it made her feel like a 'split personality'. The part played by the tutor is especially important here, as subjects of our study testified. At the academic centre each student meets her tutor in regular individual sessions.[1] It is to be expected that the relation between them will be simpler on the whole than the relation between student and supervisor, which is complicated by the work on which they are engaged together. The tutor's concern is with the student's whole process of learning. Both are aware of the ground, academic and practical, which has to be covered in the allotted period. The tutor will have to see that a student moves forward, not giving a disproportionate amount of time to some absorbing interest at the expense of subjects which those who have planned the Course consider to be im-

[1] Some of the subjects, owing to shortage of staff, shared tutorials. Occasionally, when students were ideally paired, it seems to have worked well; in other cases it was clearly a disadvantage.

portant. Yet it is also her business to ensure that the educational process builds upon the personality and past experience of each student, and follows and encourages the natural development which results from the impact of the whole Course upon the individual.

Part of the process of learning, a part which may tend to preoccupy some students at certain phases, takes place through the experience of case-work gained at the practical training centres. Here the supervisor shares with the student the actual stresses of her case-work. In this setting the student may easily see her cases too exclusively in terms of personal relationship, with the client on the one hand and the supervisor on the other. It will often happen, however, that she will bring up for discussion with her tutor cases upon which she is working and discussing week by week with her supervisor. This may be because her mind is occupied with a difficult case at the time of her tutorial, or because one of her cases illustrates some general theme which is engaging her attention in her academic study. In either case a problem, which at the practical training centre may appear chiefly one of personal relationship and of success or failure in developing professional skill, in discussion with the tutor may come to take its place in the whole volume of the student's accumulating knowledge. If the case has been a source of distress to her, she may return to the centre better able, in the light of more intellectual understanding, to handle her emotional attitudes. The tutor's general familiarity with the work of the training centres, and the constant informal interchange between tutor and supervisor, puts her in a position to help the student to think clearly about her cases without intervening in the actual process of supervision. This delicate balance between tutor and supervisor may, of course, be disturbed. Provided, however, that the members of the training staff themselves feel committed to a common purpose of learning, in their own province of student training, the advantages of this dual system greatly outweigh, in our opinion, the stresses for which it is sometimes responsible.

One might perhaps say that one of the tutor's functions is to prevent the training from turning in upon itself. It is very easy for psychiatric social case-work to become so absorbing to those who practice it that the reason for undertaking it is no longer questioned. This tendency can to some extent be met in advance through the work of the tutor who, representing the wide field of theoretical inquiry, will not allow the student to evade the task of relating what she is practising and studying with sociological and philosophical issues and facing some of the ethical considerations of the profession she has chosen.

There is another way in which the presence of the tutor may help to ease some of the problems of supervision. It is obviously unfortunate if a particular student does not work easily with a particular tutor, but any serious incompatibility between student and supervisor is likely to be yet more unfortunate. The few months spent at a training centre hardly allow such a problem of relationship to be worked through. Nor is it usually possible, even if it were desirable, for a student to be transferred to another supervisor. The best that can be hoped for is that the student so placed may be able to go on quietly learning through her case-work, with the minimum of dependence upon her supervisor. But it needs a very unusual student to be able to deal with the situation as objectively as this, and even for such a one there is likely to be some degree of loss. When incompatibility does exist, it is an important fact that no student is related to the training staff through one of its members alone. She will experience the supervision of at least two successive supervisors, while, all the time, in the greater detachment of the academic setting, the relationship of tutor and student is maintained.

It would seem that academic work, as reflected in the tutorial, is rarely satisfactory when practical work is running a disturbed course. Yet our study showed how variously the two are related. An older subject, for example, who continued to find tutorials 'a misery', showed increasing confidence and skill in her practical work. Another, who was beginning to regard her own intellectualism as a snare to her, treated her tutor 'with a certain wariness', while showing steady and outstanding progress in case-work. Constructive use of tutorials is certainly not dependent mainly upon previous educational advantages. In some cases it would seem that lack of opportunities for academic learning, in students with lively intelligence and an interest in ideas, has brought them to the tutorial especially ready and anxious to make full use of it.

A characteristic feature of the Course during the period under review was the preparation of a paper on an individually chosen subject for discussion at a seminar. This attempt to seek an answer to a limited question, while it did not entail any formal training in research, introduced students to some of the problems involved in discovery. Moreover, the presentation of the paper and the discussion which followed afforded practice in the communication of knowledge and ideas which is an important part of a social worker's equipment. The study made it clear, however, that while this form of learning met the needs of certain students admirably, others might have used the time thus spent more profitably in other ways. It could not, in any case, take the place of free discussion in classes, and an ideal Course would certainly find a place for both.[1]

As we suggested, the joint concern of supervisor and student in case-work throws into relief their own relationship—a natural result of the educational situation. Yet we were struck in our study by the widely different importance which supervision had in the memory of different subjects. For some the essence of the practical training lay simply in the experience in case-work which it offered them. We have no reason to doubt that these students made good use of all the opportunities for consultation open to them, but for them the case was the thing. One of them recalled clearly, thirteen years after her training, certain cases which had been for her 'immensely educative'. This however is a small group compared with those who regarded supervision as itself a significant experience, even when they were critical of the way it was carried out. One student from the distinction group described it as the most valuable part of the training, as well as the most full of strain. This touches the question of the essentially educational nature of this training and the importance of distinguishing it from therapy. It will already be clear, and we easily concede, that in any individual case the two are not easy to keep apart and serious mistakes may be made if this is attempted in the wrong way or for the wrong reasons. The chapter on 'Personal Difficulties' provides further material for discussion.

Up to now we have taken the presence of a supervisor of practical work for granted. Yet it might be asked why a student who is able to discuss with her tutor problems arising out of her own case-work and who at the practical training centre will be in touch

[1] An interesting comparison of the two methods by someone who knew the Course both as student and tutor, and had experience of both methods, is found in a paper by L. A. Shaw, entitled 'Groups in Education', *British Journal of Psychiatric Social Work*, 3, Nov. 1949, pp. 24–35. The emphasis here on what happens in a group, rather than upon an individual's private adventures in learning, represents a contemporary trend of interest.

with the various social workers practising their profession there, should need the regular help of a supervisor of her own, on whose time she feels she has, within understood limits, the right to draw. The first point to be considered is that of selection of cases. It is possible to be too selective in the choice of students' cases, yet it is unlikely that the time at their disposal at any centre will ever be long enough to allow for many experiments and mistakes. The needs of each student are individual, and the cases assigned to her must follow the line of her development in training, which can only be known to someone whose business it is to observe it. The supervisor herself should be fully aware of the needs of the clinic or hospital and should help the student to realize them increasingly as training advances, but these needs ought not to be the chief consideration in building up a student's experience of case-work, as we believe they would tend to be if cases were allotted to her by workers who had not been assigned a specifically educational rôle.

To most students moreover, at least in the earlier part of their time in a training centre, the work going on around them seems complicated and confusing. Even those who have previously held responsible posts now feel themselves at a disadvantage and are often exaggeratedly conscious of their ignorance. Many students find it very difficult to consult busy members of the staff about any except definite or limited questions directly arising out of their cases. If there were no person to whom they felt able to turn on any point in this new experience which they found puzzling at the moment, many would carry round with them a load of comparatively simple problems, which discussion at the right time might have helped them, if not to solve, at least to see in better proportion. To give to a period of supervision the necessary sense of leisure is hardly possible except when supervision is recognized in clinic or hospital as a definite and important duty and when the supervisor is, for the time being, sufficiently freed from other responsibilities to make herself completely available to the student and her educational needs.[1]

In the periods of discussion of case-work between student and

[1] We believe that students gain by being placed together in groups in special centres, rather than singly or by twos and threes, as is often done in providing practical experience for students of university courses in social science, when of course there may be no choice in the matter. Among the advantages is the greater likelihood that a specially planned and varied training will be provided for the larger group and that their right to educational treatment will be respected at the place of training.

supervisor a number of educational processes take place. It is an important fact that, when a case has been referred to a student, the supervisor, although she will have various ways of following its general progress, can only know through the student herself what takes place in the interviews between her and the client. This is brought sharply home if, as may occasionally happen, the supervisor is forced to doubt the reliability of the reports of some student who cannot resist dramatizing or putting the best complexion upon the part she herself has played in an interview. But if the supervisor's dependence on the student in this sense can sometimes be an embarrassment, it has also a high educational value. There is thrown upon the student the responsibility of making the supervisor realize, either by oral or written reporting, the people, relations, situations and problems which go to make up the case, and what her intervention in it has meant. It is one of the most satisfying experiences in supervision to note how a meagre and lifeless account, in which the narrator seems to have seen very little significance, becomes vital and full of meaning for the student herself as she is led on to unfold to the supervisor impressions which she has actually received during the interview but has not known what to do with.

Some students are, from the beginning, very much alive to their own part in the interplay of case-work. For a few this interest may become excessive, but many others, among them some of the most promising, need to have their attention held to this matter and to be led to value the comparative leisure of the training period as an opportunity for studying what happens in the case-work process. To watch with students and help them to strike a balance between an artificial concentration upon their own part in cases and a failure to examine it at all is one of the tasks of the supervisor which depends upon continuity in supervision.

The student who is only led with difficulty to recognize her own part in case-work may well be one who finds the responsibility of it hard to accept. This responsibility should in discussion with a supervisor become less overwhelming, and may indeed somewhat change its character as the student is helped to understand what psychiatric social work can and cannot hope to achieve. The possibilities and the limitations of this work can be kept before a student's notice, so that every new case will add to her appreciation of the problem, as something about which the profession as a whole is seeking to think more clearly.

When the relation between them is sound, a student can be helped to use her supervisor to recognize such stereotyped ideas as may have been unwittingly forming in her mind of certain figures in her case-work, such as the step-mother or the adolescent in revolt, or relationships and situations to which she tends to react in stereotyped ways. It is for the supervisor to be alive to the possibility of such compulsive thinking, which the student cannot easily recognize unaided, since it is likely to be rooted in the less accessible levels of personal development. The revealing of such stereotypes, as they seem to be operating in a student's case-work, does not necessarily involve the interpretation of their origins; for this indeed most supervisors would not feel themselves adequately equipped.

It has sometimes been asked whether a student training to become a psychiatric social worker would not profit by sitting-in at interviews between her supervisor and a client. We believe that most psychiatric social workers would turn down the suggestion, but it is important to consider on what grounds. We ourselves see two main objections. The first concerns the welfare of the client. In any interview which is in the nature of treatment, where the relationship between worker and client is essential for the task to be carried out between them, it is hard to believe that the presence of a third person would not seriously hinder the process. But while it is recognized that there is no kind of interview in which the relations between client and worker is not important, we can conceive that an experienced worker, at ease with herself, could introduce a student into certain kinds of interviews without damage to the client. The other objection concerns the student's training. When it is suggested that a student would profit by 'listening in' to an experienced worker, it is presumably thought of as a means of hastening the growth of skill in building up a relationship and of working with a client towards self-understanding and release. The obvious time to introduce such an aid to learning would seem to be at the earlier stage, when the student feels particularly inadequate and unsure of herself. Yet such a stage is a necessary one and a short cut is educationally unsound. The student's need is rather of help in tolerating her own discomfort, perhaps for quite a long time. An experienced worker will have her own way of playing her part in an interview, which, if it is sincere, will be the reflection of her own personality. To an insecure student, however, this may appear as a technique which she can adopt, whether it is an authentic expression of her own personality or not. Perhaps one might say paradoxically that it would only be safe, as an educational method, for a student to be present when her supervisor is interviewing, when she no longer feels the need to do so and is no longer tempted to snatch at another's technique.[1]

At a later stage a student might obviously profit from being present at certain kinds of interviews between an experienced worker and a client. There are many other things to learn besides the fundamental skill to which we have just referred. Several subjects spoke of how much they had learned from visiting with an experienced visitor in mental deficiency. The educational aim of such visits was limited, viz., to open up and make real to the student the nature of mental deficiency, its special problems and the provisions made to meet them, not to train her to become an expert in this branch of mental welfare.

In the training for work with adults, students attend clinical conferences where patients are introduced, and also sit in with psychiatrists at out-patient clinics. They thus reap the benefit of a way of learning which has its roots in medical education. Since we knew that students were sometimes considerably disturbed by this during their training, we raised the point with most of the subjects whom we interviewed. The general opinion was that, for the learning of psychiatry, this method had been very helpful indeed. On the whole, as one might have expected, this fact seemed to overshadow in their memory the anxiety which some of them undoubtedly felt at the time over the effect on patients of this way of learning. One spoke of having been disturbed by it at first, but of having been able to 'switch over to an attitude of inquiry'. The point on which there was general agreement was that the way in which the psychiatrist handled the situation was all important.

Students of the Mental Health Course have to accept the fact that they are heavily indebted to those patients and relatives at whose expense they gain their knowledge and skill. Many have been

[1] A subject of our study, who has herself had experience in the practical training of students, raised an interesting point. About the danger of adopting, through listening to interviews, a technique not suited to one's own temperament, she suggested that some students do this whether they hear others interview or not. 'We get a mental image of what we imagine a psychiatric interview to be from those who tutor us. The identification or projection is there at first whatever the conditions. . . . I don't think "listening in" to another psychiatric social worker at work, if she can let you, is more liable to identification —not with a person but with a technique—than the fantasy one gets.'

troubled by the responsibility of learning through their own casework. One student seemed less aware of this. She wrote: 'I feel that there is too much supervision in relation to the amount of practice and material. One had not the opportunity of reaching independently a state of interested curiosity or of discovering where one most needed help. I think that one could have been left to flounder more freely, without damage to the patients, and to the great advantage of one's training.' This is surely to treat a serious responsibility too lightly.

In the course of our study, more than one psychiatrist referee expressed the view that students of the Mental Health Course were too dependent for their training upon the supervision of psychiatric social workers and had too little practice in working with psychiatrists. From the subjects themselves we have some material which bears on this point. We asked most of those whom we interviewed whether as students they had been able to obtain the necessary discussion with psychiatrists on the cases on which they were working, especially at the centre of adult training, where, for various reasons, this had never been easy to achieve. On the whole the position as the students remembered it cannot be regarded as satisfactory. In some cases it was a matter of 'small expectations'. An almoner student always took it for granted that a doctor would be in a hurry, and certain of the notably weaker students were evidently content simply to receive from the psychiatrist instructions about the social measures to be taken. This would have been quite unsatisfactory to students who were experienced social workers. A very able subject of this class complained that the psychiatrists, when she consulted them about her cases, were always 'teaching at' her. It was noticeable, however, at the time, and was borne out by the evidence of the study, that there were students of many different types who did overcome the difficulties and achieved, even at the centre for work with adults, real consultation with psychiatrists over their cases. Even among those who made a general complaint most could point to some psychiatrist as a 'shining exception'. It is natural that a student of the Mental Health Course, undergoing training in work with adults in a psychiatric institution, should be very much aware of her own lack of knowledge, more aware than in a child guidance clinic where the emphasis is less medical. Several subjects admitted that their attempts to discuss their cases with the psychiatrist had been rather half-hearted, and that they were quite glad not to have to expose their own ignorance. One added that in any case she 'always had her supervisor'.

The value of co-operation between psychiatrist and psychiatric social worker depends much upon the extent to which each understands and respects the other's contribution. They need moreover to learn to work together, a question which is considered again in the chapter called 'Working in Partnership'. This cannot begin too early. The student of the Mental Health Course benefits by learning to work with those in process of becoming psychiatrists, but most of all with psychiatrists with wisdom based on experience. Through discussion with such a psychiatrist of cases on which they are both working she will learn much that cannot be conveyed through lectures or demonstrations, and much beside formal psychiatry.

We sympathize with the psychiatrist referee who finds very irksome 'the kind of exhibitionism which shows itself in a desire for unnecessary consultations and prolonged discussions over trivial matters'. It is not this that we are advocating. Some psychiatric social workers have no doubt lacked discretion and some may have been tempted to magnify the importance of their cases because they were theirs. It is during the training period that professional discretion and a sense of proportion have to be learned, and any means by which psychiatrist and psychiatric social workers are brought together in real pooling of experience and ideas during this time should contribute to this end, and the benefit should not be one-sided. After qualification the student will be working with psychiatrists of various standpoints and degrees of wisdom and experience; she needs to learn during training to appreciate the problems this involves. While we believe that casework supervision by a supervisor who is herself a psychiatric social worker has no satisfactory substitute, we also recognize that students may be too dependent upon her. To this there can be no better antidote than for them to work in increasingly close association with psychiatrists who themselves appreciate the special nature and problems of the profession for which the students are preparing.[1]

During most of the period of which we have been writing, students had some experience of a third place of practical training—

[1] This is a strong argument for 'team training' in clinical practice, though not, in our view, for separating psychiatric social workers from the centres of study of social sciences, where they have their roots.

a mental observation ward.[1] It was upon this subsidiary training that they commented most freely and, as a rule, most appreciatively. It would appear that the relatively small size of the unit, the unmistakable reality of the problems that faced them there, the way in which students were accepted into the unit as working members all combined to give a number of them satisfaction which they did not find in either of the other centres. Some spoke of what they had gained from working closely alongside the psychiatric social workers concerned. One learned much from observing the quick handling of critical situations and of seeing the general reliance placed upon the social worker and how she 'pulled things together'. One felt more at home here than in the larger adult centre because she was more part of the job and less of a student, while another, to whom up to then psychiatry had been 'something outside herself', found that at the observation ward it 'came alive'.

There is a certain kind of learning which is likely to occur irrespective of the conditions in which the more formal learning takes place, though some are more favourable to it than others. We refer to the unplanned education of students through the student group. What her group meant to her is described in a report from a student for whom special arrangements had to be made, so that she always felt out of step with the rest. 'Contact with other students was the most stimulating and valuable experience of training. They had such widely varying backgrounds, personalities, temperaments and gifts. I remember still the long discussions over endless cups of tea and cigarettes and am glad that, even with all the work we had to do, there was still time for these sessions. . . . It was a disadvantage to start my practical training four months after the other members of my year. . . . I was on the outside of the group and was rather surprised to find how much I wanted to be accepted by it.' For some students the value of the group lay chiefly in mental stimulation and the sharing of intellectual discovery, to others it meant emotional support. Several subjects spoke of how, when their work in child guidance led to the revival of their own early memories, they were able to keep a sense of proportion through finding in discussions among the group that others were going through the same experience.

It seemed to us significant that those non-qualified subjects with

[1] A unit, not in a mental hospital, where in urgent cases a mentally ill person can, under the Lunacy Act of 1890, be detained without a Justice's order for not longer than seventeen days.

whom this matter was discussed did not seem to have been at ease in their groups. One spoke of having felt 'inhibited' in a group which she regarded as outstanding in intelligence and personality. One had little contact with other students as a whole, though an older student 'jollied her along'. Another was irritated by the way her fellow students 'wasted their time', 'like a lot of hilarious school girls'.[1] It would seem that this subject had not been able to appreciate one function of the group which seems to us of some importance—the light relief which it can afford in a training all too liable to overwhelm some individuals with its seriousness, by helping to preserve, towards theories and people alike, a certain amused detachment.

It was noticeable too that these unqualified subjects had little to say about the training as a whole. It would seem that they were too much concerned with their own difficulties as students to view it at all objectively. Our inquiries about the way their personal difficulties had been handled by the staff brought a few comments, of which the most important were in answer to the question whether they 'felt that they should have been given, as they went along, a more honest assessment of their work'. One subject thought that she should have been given much clearer reasons why her work was regarded as unsatisfactory. She believed that she was always open to criticism and would have honestly tried to make use of it, but when she asked 'why?' the answer was never clear enough to act upon. It is inevitable that these situations should appear somewhat differently to the training staff. As we try to show in a later chapter, there are sometimes valid reasons for being slow to give a student a general assessment of her work when it is not going well, although one might expect the weekly discussion of her cases to warn her that her suitability for psychiatric social work is open to question. It seems, however, that some students, especially those who have been eager to be admitted to the Course and convinced in advance of their suitability for the work, are unable to accept the criticism which they receive from their supervisors on individual cases as indicating a general doubt.

One of us remembers a student whose work she had to criticize week by week so seriously that she feared that confidence would be

[1] Adolescent behaviour among students as a group, even when they were mature and experienced, has often been noticed in the Mental Health Course. It is, indeed, a matter of common observation among students faced with work which makes great demands on their sympathy and responsible judgment.

altogether undermined. When, however, the final unfavourable assessment was discussed with her she declared that she was completely unprepared for it. This was clearly bad supervision. We do not think that this student could, in any case, have been helped to make good use of the training, but the supervisor should have realized her inability to grasp the general implications of the detailed weekly criticism. It is interesting to find that the same may apply to appreciation. A subject whose work was held in high esteem throughout the Course, and who was finally awarded a mark of distinction, declared that it would have helped her greatly if she had been made to realize during training that her work was regarded as good. To have been told this had not been enough. It is possible that in psychiatric social work, where sensitiveness to the feelings of others is professionally cultivated, supervisors sometimes overstep the mark and fall into the habit of approaching students' educational problems in too indirect and implicit a manner, failing to convey the impression which is so clear in their own minds and at times arousing anxiety when they intend to reassure.

One may distinguish two processes which run through professional training, that of helping the student to learn and that of assessing her capacity to use the particular training on which she has embarked. The distinction is really artificial, since the student's progress in learning can be greatly influenced by the way tutor or supervisor withholds from her or conveys to her the assessment which she has reached. Assessment, of course, goes on throughout the whole learning process. In the short and exacting training which we have described, and with the variety which exists among the students, it has not been customary to arrange for formal assessments of the students' work at frequent intervals. There is little enough time for the seed to grow without disturbing it more often than is strictly necessary. Yet it is obviously not in the mind of the training staff alone that the process of assessment goes on; in the mind of the student also, more or less consciously, a parallel process is taking place. Some of those who did not qualify evidently felt that here indeed were lines which would never meet.

iii

If we were asked to say what the Mental Health Course ought to have given to a student by the end of training, both as a general educational process and as a preparation for psychiatric social work, we could enumerate certain kinds of equipment with which it should have provided her. We could mention a body of knowledge; an understanding, made real through direct work with people, of certain principles underlying human behaviour and human relations; experience of how to use her own equipment as a social worker in association with psychiatry; skill in the professional use of relationship and of her own personality in a disciplined professional way. Yet such a list, we suspect, would not seem to those who had passed through the training to get very near to its essential nature.

The kind of work which the social worker does and the fact that she herself forms part of the social field which it is her concern to study are not conducive to drawing a sharp line between professional and personal. We found how inextricably the two were bound up when we asked the subjects of our study two questions; one about the way their training had affected them personally and the other about the means by which, after they had qualified, they had added to their professional understanding and skill. With a large proportion of subjects the replies to these two questions could not be kept apart. A common type of answer was that training had given a degree of new understanding, which was then applied to personal experience and sometimes modified by it; such understanding would then flow back into professional experience with greater depth and realism. We shall therefore consider the answers to both questions in the present chapter.

The statement 'I think it would be impossible to do the training and remain unaffected personally' seems to represent the opinion of most of those who answered the first of these questions. The wide-reaching effect of the training upon a very young student was described in a way which emphasizes the Course's responsibility in admitting anyone, however brilliant, at a very malleable phase. 'The questions I was asking in 1932 (her student year) were answered in a large measure in certain terms, using a certain vocabulary, and certain keys of interpretation, as a result of taking the Mental Health Course—being still in a very developing stage, it was all incorporated from the start in my emotional growth and understanding.' It would be misleading to suggest that this represents the usual response to training. Most students, entering the Course with a variety of experience behind them, while agreeing that the Course had not left them as it found them in personal development, accepted this additional experience as part of the wider flow of life. We have heard it suggested that it is desirable to admit students young to the mental health courses, because they are then still 'malleable'. There is something disturbing in this suggestion; its implications, in any case, call for the most careful and honest scrutiny. In fact, it is not our experience that the younger students are necessarily the more malleable; some are well able to resist the pressure of persons and ideas. Yet defensiveness is a pitiful substitute for the readiness to learn (a very different thing from malleability) which characterizes true maturity.

Two subjects certainly expressed a fear of being turned through training from their natural bent. Most, however, seem to have welcomed change, while recognizing that it must entail some loss, not necessarily permanent, such as diminished spontaneity and confidence in their own intuitions. Some, who reported on the greater general detachment which they had gained through training, denied that increased understanding of the springs of behaviour had changed their attitudes to family or friends, and a few added, with great emphasis, that they hoped it never would. Several attributed to their training a growing tolerance. While a few seemed to fear this, as though it might proceed so far that their own personalities would become disintegrated, to most it evidently meant a welcome release. One now saw herself as overconfident at the end of training and foolishly 'superior', a state often apparent to certain critics of psychiatric social workers, whose criticisms we shall consider in a later chapter.

In connexion with the second of the two questions we provided a list[1] of eleven possible sources of increase in professional understanding and skill since training and asked the subjects to mark those which applied to them. It seemed to us significant that in the distinction group there was a comparatively high proportion of those who attributed their professional development to a large number of sources. We shall consider two of these. The first has remained in psychiatric social work since her qualification sixteen years ago. She attributes her development to her professional experience and research, to her professional association, to 'sporadic' study and general reading and to travel for professional purposes. She has also learned, she suggests, through 'parenthood at second-

[1] This comprised professional experience, the professional association, help of colleagues, systematic study and other reading, travel for professional purposes, marriage and parenthood and other personal experiences.

hand', by way of a crowd of nephews, nieces and god-children; and, finally, by 'just growing older'. The second is married and has children. Because of family responsibilities she has not been able to undertake more than temporary full-time work as a psychiatric social worker, but has engaged in a wide range of part-time work, much of it educational, in which her training has been turned to good account. The only sources of professional development which she did not mark were those from which, at least in part, she was debarred by her way of life, viz., systematic study, research and travel for professional purposes. Personal analysis, with marriage and parenthood, was marked as especially important. The impression made by her list is confirmed by the independent comment of one of her referees, that she had the capacity for using personal experience in her professional work to an unusual degree.

When we studied the responses to the different possible sources of development which we suggested, some interesting facts emerged. As was to be expected nearly every subject marked 'Professional experience', the accumulated gain of just going on with one's job; one paid tribute in passing to what she had learned from the mothers with whom she worked at a child guidance clinic. 'Help from colleagues' came next in the score. Nearly half counted membership of their professional association as a source of professional development. This is not as high a proportion as one might have expected, but, as one subject remarked, 'one gets more from an association when one works for it', and among our subjects, as among the membership in general, it is a small number only upon whose shoulders the work of the Association has always rested. It is perhaps more difficult to explain why several who have rendered the association much service, did not mark it as a source of professional growth. Very few indeed referred to 'systematic study'; many on the other hand referred to reading though, not unnaturally, they often found it difficult to give off-hand the names of books which had been important to them.

Of the personal sources of development on our list, 'marriage' and 'parent-hood' did not lead to any comments, but 'other types of personal experience' brought varied responses. We noted a tendency to fear professional narrowness. One subject remarked on the value of associating with social workers who were not 'psychiatric', and one of living among people who represented many different kinds of life. This point is put most forcibly by a married subject who wrote of the importance of 'contact with a world alien to psychiatric work, e.g., the Regular Army, invaluable in making one appreciate the need and positive value of discipline.' She went on to stress the importance of 'travel *not* professional' and contact with other civilizations. Some were aware of using all personal experience in their professional work, 'from forming relationships to change in social attitudes around—to odd things like a play or a chance coincidence or happening.' One wrote of 'experience in practising a religion'; others of 'getting older'. Another, comprehensively, wrote 'Life'!

In our schedule, one of the possible sources of professional development was a personal analysis. We included this because some psychiatric social workers, and some of the clinicians with whom they work, regard this experience as educationally illuminating, if not essential to the work which they are expecting to undertake. In U.S.A. this view is much more widely held. This 'source' was marked by seventeen out of the sixty-five subjects who answered the question. Further information about the analysis was not asked for, although it was sometimes given in this or another connexion. One subject was well advanced in an analysis when she entered training; in the case of another it was the training which had given her the 'courage' to undertake one; others took this step some time after the end of training. Others again were considering the question of an analysis, but up to the time of the interview had not been able to reach a decision or had not so far been able to afford it. Their reason for wishing for an analysis was either that they recognized that unresolved personal problems were obtruding into their professional life or that they hoped by this means to fit themselves for more intensive case-work.

We do not ourselves hold the view that a personal analysis is an indispensable qualification for psychiatric social work, nor that the contribution which those who have been analysed are able to make to their profession is necessarily greater than that made by colleagues who have undergone no analysis. But while we do not regard it as one of the hall-marks of a psychiatric social worker, we should expect a personal analysis for some workers to lead to increased insight in carrying out their own work. It seems to us important to differentiate between increased insight and the lessening of tension resulting from a successful analysis which could hardly fail to benefit any professional work (not least the kind we are discussing). The advisability of undertaking an analysis will depend both on considerations of personality and of the level at which a particular worker wishes to carry out her work. In the case of some workers it would seem that what is gained through analysis may be paid for by some narrowing of range. The question of the stage at which an analysis is best undertaken is a very individual matter. Only in the case of exceptional people does it seem wise for students to be undergoing any form of sustained psychotherapy while they are under training, since such treatment is hardly compatible with the degree of self-discipline which the Course inevitably demands. The situation is different when, as in training for play-therapy, the analysis is recognized as part of the training itself.

Our study brought us criticisms of the London Mental Health Course as a preparation for psychiatric social work. It will have become clear that the Course is not regarded as a training which prepares students in detail for specific posts in their profession. The wide scope of the training and the variety of posts to be found within psychiatric social work, as well as the developments taking place there, would make this impossible. Nevertheless, it is important that training and employment should be frequently measured the one against the other, so that any unnecessary discrepancies between them may be adjusted. We shall consider here what seems to us the most important of the criticisms, whether they come from subjects or referees. Most of these represent, from various points of view, the opinion that the conditions of training have been too artificial or specialized to form an adequate introduction to the realities of employment, as students will meet them in the field. With regard to adult work the emphasis is on the lack of experience in the grosser forms of mental illness and in the conditions of a general as compared with a specialized mental hospital. With regard to child guidance the criticism is less specific, referring to a somewhat artificial atmosphere and an excessive concentration upon problems of intensive case-work, at the expense of an introduction to questions of administration and of the clinic's relations with the community which it serves.

Many of these points, and some others with which we have already dealt, are brought together in a report from a referee in a child guidance clinic. He writes: 'It seems that during the Course, their previous confidence in relation to their rôle of social worker is broken down, but that they have not yet acquired a new approach and security in its place. It seems that they are still over-dependent on their tutors and seem to have had too little opportunity for doing more case-work under decreasing supervision but with a supporting background. I consequently find that they need quite intensive teaching continued from the psychiatrist during the first 12 months. . . . I wonder if they have adequate opportunity of seeing the potentialities of C.G. service as a Community Service and of seeing it function prophylactically? Most of their work is done in London clinics where the work has a 'hospital' trend and the full community links of a C.G. service, so essential in the Provinces, do not seem to be developed. . . . Again, they seem to have little knowledge of the 'local authority mind' and how to cope with it without becoming either frustrated or aggressive! This also is something they have no direct experience of during training and will be the most important thing they will have to cope with afterwards unless working at a hospital.'

It should be mentioned that during the final month of training (recently increased to two) a considerable proportion of students have sought experience in provincial clinics as well as in county mental hospitals. But this has never been compulsory and many have remained at their training centres, consolidating their experience in long-term case-work for which, it is true, the time is all too short. Some of the subjects have suggested that the training should gradually be made to approximate, as far as this can be arranged, to the far from perfect conditions students are likely to find in their jobs, so that they may be helped to distinguish, as part of their training, how far to adjust themselves to conditions they find there, and how far and in what way, to make a serious attempt to modify them. One subject suggested that students would be helped if, towards the end of training, members of the staff shared with them more frankly than they do their own knowledge of difficulties ahead, especially in pioneer jobs. A referee with wide experience in community service emphasized the importance of helping students to understand where the psychiatric social worker's special responsibility lies when a case is carried cooperatively with social workers without psychiatric training.

One of the subjects, speaking of general tendencies in training in her day, suggested that there was a danger of learning to become 'a good student rather than a good psychiatric social worker.' This is a serious criticism of a professional training. It is certainly true that we came upon a group of five who did not seem, according to their referees, to be fulfilling the expectations which their careers as students had aroused. To say that they were 'good students' but not 'good psychiatric social workers' would do them much less than justice. All have useful work to their credit and several have held, with apparent success, posts of special importance and difficulty; yet their achievement in employment has shown limitations or signs of stress which do not appear to have been foreseen in their student days. On the other hand we found a much larger group whose record in employment exceeded the promise of their student years. We propose to consider these two groups in the chapter that follows, which aims at illustrating the various ways in which careers after qualification work themselves out.

CHAPTER VI

THE SHAPING OF CAREERS

i

PURSUING the suggestion that the Mental Health Course tends to produce good students rather than good psychiatric social workers, we begin this chapter with a study of the five subjects, out of the forty-two on whom we were able to obtain an assessment from psychiatrist referees, in whose case the expectations of the training period do not seem to have been altogether fulfilled in employment. In age from 24 to 45, they entered the Course very differently equipped. The eldest was a social worker of considerable experience, while two came from other professions and had gained their experience in social work chiefly through voluntary service. Three held university degrees but only one held a social science certificate. At selection one was regarded as a very doubtful candidate and only one was assessed highly. Did the good level of achievement during training, in all but one case above the expectations at selection, indicate a real gain, which for some reason was not maintained, or was the apparent gain a reflection of the artificial conditions of training, which did not lead to genuine professional growth?

Seeking for any factors which might have caused these five subjects to show at their best in training, we noticed that all were intellectually competent and found much satisfaction in the academic side of the Course. Several entered with keen expectations; one felt that she had at last found what she had been groping for. None seemed unduly disturbed during training. It is true that reports mention certain difficulties, for example, lack of confidence, and, in two cases, immaturity, yet these were evidently not regarded as marked enough to constitute serious handicaps. Several, when we interviewed them for the study, told spontaneously of how much they had enjoyed their time as students.

The opening phase of their careers as psychiatric social workers contained a common feature which may be significant—none had the advantage of consolidating their original training by drawing upon the experience of senior colleagues. One, who obtained a post in a fully staffed child guidance clinic, found the conditions of work there generally unfortunate and the psychiatric social worker already established there unable to help her because of her own personal difficulties. Another accepted an important post under the impression that she was to work as an assistant but found that in fact she was to work alone. In two cases the organization did not include a psychiatrist.

In the period between the first post and the post to which the psychiatrists' reports apply we find, on the limited information at our disposal, no common features which appear significant. It is to the reports of the psychiatrist referees themselves, in three cases supported in a general sense by a second referee,[1] to which we must trust for light upon this discrepancy between achievement in training and employment. In fact there runs through these reports a hint of a common feature, which seems best described as uneasiness in regard to one's own aggressive tendencies. This may appear in case-work as a fear of going below the surface. One subject to whom this kind of superficiality is ascribed is referred to as 'nice and lady-like' and as having her aggression well in control. In another the situation is different. This subject is said to be increasingly capable of 'quite deep and intensive case-work' but to continue to have difficulties with colleagues inside and outside her clinic, so that she has gained an undeserved reputation for officiousness. The difficulties in relationship experienced by subjects range from office staff to administrative superior. The problem which authority presents to them is illustrated clearly in two cases. In the first the subject is described as at her best when in charge, but going to pieces in the face of obstruction and criticism. The second wanted a senior post, yet felt inferior when it came to her and had not the knack of being in charge without making others aware of it. With a third subject the position is comparable but the stress falls upon ambition. She is described as 'striving for success and public acknowledgment of her capabilities', and often 'overreaching herself'.

In this group of able students, all of whom regard psychiatric social work as the work for which they are best suited, achievement

[1] It was not possible in two instances to get the views of a second referee.

in the work of their choice is interfered with by difficulties in relationship. In some cases this has affected their case-work; in all it has tended to make their dealings with those they work with uncertain and strained. It may be assumed that their own aggression presented problems to all of them, not least to the one who is said to have had hers under control and at the same time to have kept to the surface in case-work. Driven back to look more closely at the training period and to ask whether there was really no trace of this kind of difficulty there, we can only reply that nothing of the kind is reported, either in case-work, in relations with the training staff or with colleagues inside or outside the practical training centres. We remember, it is true, how one of the older subjects showed a deference to the opinions of her supervisor, in matters in which she was in fact the more experienced of the two, which suggested at the time aggressive feeling too tightly held in control. Yet this was conjecture only. Others of the group are described as diffident or lacking in ease, yet within normal limits. It would seem then that the conditions of the training obscured traits which were to appear later and were not such as to make these particular students turn and face their difficulties. Among these conditions may be the relaxation which comes from being a student again, the support of the student group, the satisfaction for intellectually able students arising from all the academic aspects of the Course. In the case of these students after-events suggest that their problems were shelved and not solved.

The existence of even so small a proportion whose achievement in employment does not seem to have fulfilled the expectations of the training period is disquieting. We must admit that greater perceptiveness and skill on the part of the training staff might have brought into the open latent difficulties, which the student could then have been helped to face within the protected conditions of training. A more determined effort, as the training draws to a close, to bring these conditions closer to those of actual employment, where she is no longer an object of educational concern, might provide more situations in which a student's aggressive tendencies would be called out. Within the Course the effects of these upon others would be less disturbing than in employment, and would be accepted as part of learning and growing. Yet we should not expect any comprehensive and lasting solution of these students' problems within a short educational course; our impression is that in all these cases the problems were profound and deeply embedded in the personality. Their existence has not prevented those who carry them from playing a useful part in psychiatric social work, but it is not surprising to find that three of the five have had recourse to a personal analysis. None show that complacency which is the only fatal enemy to growth.

ii

Less disturbing is the existence of a group of eleven subjects who, at the time when our study caught them, were apparently doing better in their posts than their achievement as students had given reason to expect. That this group is more than twice as large as that of students who seem to have been over-estimated reminds one of the tendency to under-estimate found in selection. We had to admit the possibility that the tendency in that phase had led to the rejection of some candidates who would in fact have proved suitable for training. In the same way the discovery of under-estimation during training suggests that some of those who were advised to withdraw before the end of the Course, or were failed by the Board of Examiners, might have made good in employment. Nevertheless, in view of the prolonged and careful consideration which always precedes the advice to withdraw, and, in the case of those who sat for examinations, of the number of independent opinions represented by the Board, such misjudgments are likely to have been rare.

Keeping in mind the characteristics of the group we have just considered, we shall look at some of the more significant features of these eleven subjects. The number of graduates is small, three only, though two have had a broken period at a university. All but one, however, hold a social science certificate, a proportion considerably larger than for the subjects of our study as a whole. The proportion of those who have held responsible posts in some branch of social work before admission is also high. With regard to age, one might expect a group which did better in employment than in training to include a large proportion of those who found it difficult to accept the position of student and these we might reasonably look for among candidates who entered the Course at a comparatively late age. But the ages of the eleven subjects do not bear this out. All except two fall within the span of 25 to 35, usually regarded as the most suitable for entering, and the exceptions only deviate, one at each end, by a couple of years.

There is evidence, however, that several members of this group did, for various reasons, find it difficult to adjust themselves to the training. In one case temperament and previous experience seem to have been the chief causes; two others found the system of individual teaching characteristic of the Course so different from anything they had experienced before that they could not easily make use of it. A few were personally disturbed during their training; two of them undertook a personal analysis at a later period. One, who found the Course a tiring one and made a somewhat negative impression at this time, was found later to have been suffering from a physical condition which is likely to have prevented her as a student from showing her full capacity and which has since been satisfactorily treated. On the whole we should say that this group enjoyed their training less than the last and showed less intellectual zest, although the capacity of the group was not low. It should be noted that three were returning in employment to the high assessment they were given at selection.

Recalling the experience of the previous group with regard to first posts, we note that the present group were not obviously more fortunate in opportunities to consolidate their training. It is true that on qualification one student secured a bursary and another an assistant post, but several went straight from training to their former type of work or undertook a succession of posts as *locum*, or spent a year in voluntary social work not specifically psychiatric. A feature common to most of the group is indeed this rather slow settling into a permanent post recognized as psychiatric.

We have considered elsewhere the tendency of psychiatric referees to rate their subjects high and we note that in three cases in our present group a psychiatric social worker colleague, acting as second referee, makes a somewhat lower assessment. In several cases the psychiatrist indicates that the subject is the kind of person with whom he or she likes to work, and that the assessment must be taken as a strictly personal one. It may be that this special ability of two particular people to work harmoniously together enters into the high assessment made by a psychiatrist referee of one of the subjects who was rated comparatively low both for selection and training. But this cannot be the whole explanation, and because her career raises a number of considerations which apply to others of this group, we shall discuss it at some length. At selection the impression she made on her different interviewers was not consistent and she herself seemed somewhat uncertain whether this was the right type of work for her. The doubt lingered among the staff during her training and she never seemed much at home in the Course. In case-work, while she made considerable progress, her work seems to have remained superficial. On the academic side she found it particularly difficult to make any use of her tutorials. In general she was regarded as a friendly, likeable person, but it was agreed at the end of training that she was not yet fit to undertake any but an assistant post. This she was able to obtain and enjoyed the experience. The war gave scope for work of another character, in a clinic for evacuated children, with a psychiatrist who respected her.

It is instructive to see what qualities the psychiatrist referee singles out for praise. She writes: 'I think that her success is largely to be attributed to her own essential normality. She is evidently well-balanced and this quality is reflected in her work. One never feels that her own personal problems influence it in any way and she never shows the slightest sign of jealousy over any slight infringement of her work and position. Her judgment is very sound; she knows when to press a point and when to leave it and thus she is excellent at slowly converting hostile outsiders to her point of view.' In trying to understand the discrepancies between the assessments made on this subject at the two first stages and at the third, we have to take into account what was required of her in training and in her job as her psychiatrist saw it. Here, apart from the duties of public relations officer to which our quotation refers, the emphasis is upon the production of social histories for the psychiatrist's use, on interviewing and on maintaining a good relationship with foster-parents. There is no reference to the psychiatric social worker as engaged in 'treatment', in the sense in which this term is commonly used by psychiatric social workers. In training, on the other hand, while the social history takes an important place and the need for a student to gain experience in interpreting her work to others is fully recognized, 'treatment', especially of the mother of a child patient at a child guidance clinic, is apt to be made the touchstone of the student's work.

We believe this emphasis during training to be justified, yet, on account of it, the qualities needed for such work may be too exclusively valued, at the expense of the other qualities found in this and other members of the present group, which only came to be fully appreciated when they undertook an ordinary job in the open field. Perhaps it was inevitable that conditions in a training centre should fail to draw attention to this subject's assets. In the relatively complicated situation of a supervised student doing highly responsible case-work, her rather uncomplicated personality may have seemed less clear in its aims than in fact it was, while her common sense, her lack of concern with her own status and her capacity for unobtrusive educational work may have received less than their due.

Recapitulating some of the features of the two groups which seem to us to have a possible significance, we note that in the first only one subject had the preliminary qualifications demanded by the Course with regard both to training and experience, as compared with the second where the proportion of those who had a social science certificate was unusually high. We noticed too that in the second group more of the subjects had their feet planted firmly in social work. With regard to training, the first group was probably somewhat more intellectually able than the second and got more satisfaction from the academic side of the Course. Passing over differences in the sphere of employment which are of doubtful significance, we recall the fact that difficulties in professional relationships, connected with control of aggressive tendencies, seemed to loom significantly large in the first group. In the second, where this appears at all, it seems to be confined to a much smaller area of professional life.

All the members of both groups were studied at a distance of between ten and fifteen years from the end of their training. For most we may assume at least as long a professional career ahead as that on which our study is based. What we have learned seems to offer certain suggestions and warnings to those concerned in training. There are qualities to which the artificial conditions of training do not give full play although they are in fact of great value in meeting the wider demands of a psychiatric social worker's job. These can easily be under-estimated in the student. On the other hand, qualities which may give rise to difficulties in the unprotected field of employment may be masked during training, and so not brought within the educational process. Nevertheless, we cannot be sure that the distinction between the two groups would be so clear if we were to consider the same subjects ten or fifteen years hence. The end of formal training is only the opening of a door into new experiences. It has no finality. The apparent drop in standard from training to employment, based on the assessment of particular referees, does not mean that the standard of the subjects concerned will not rise at a later period. We notice that two of this group are at present in course of a personal analysis and that the case-work of one of them is already showing the benefit. There are many circumstances which might cause any of these students to be assessed more highly at a later stage, such as conditions of work bringing out latent powers, association with a particular psychiatrist or other colleague, and a whole range of personal experience. With the other group, of course, the future is equally unpredictable.

It has sometimes been maintained that students who qualify in the Mental Health Course should be placed in classes according to merit. This is not customary in professional training and our study of these two groups illustrates how singularly unsuitable such a procedure would be in training for psychiatric social work, where qualification represents so varied a blend of achievement in training and possibilities of achievement in employment.

iii

At an earlier stage of our study we thought very largely in terms of the job which a subject happened to be holding at the time when we interviewed her. It soon became clear, however, that the meaning of a job depended for the holder upon where it stood in the sequence of employment from qualification up to the time of the interview. Having realized this we had to guard against reading too subtle a meaning into every move, and remind ourselves that a genuine wish could not always be carried out at a particular time. Someone whose main interest was child guidance might seek her first post in a mental hospital because she wanted to widen her experience before settling down to her chosen work. Another might take such a post because, at the moment when she qualified, there were no vacancies in child guidance and she could not afford to wait. We asked our subjects what 'circumstances and considerations' led them into their first post as psychiatric social workers and influenced them in changing their jobs. This formula did not necessarily uncover underlying motives, but, as we talked, these sometimes became apparent.

A newly qualified psychiatric social worker has not made a clear break with her past. A number of subjects, when they entered the Course, had behind them careers long enough for a pattern to have emerged. These were related in differing ways with the form which their careers took after training. A varied and apparently restless career before training followed by a later career marked by no more than an average amount of change, and this of a purposive kind, would suggest that in psychiatric social work a subject had at last found the work for which she was fitted. But a restless career might equally represent a fundamentally restless and adventurous temperament and we should not expect a one year's training to change this. We need not be surprised if, after such a subject leaves the Course, she passes from one post to another within psychiatric social work and perhaps, in the end, passes outside it. Our material gives us examples of both.

At the end of the chapter we give tables illustrating the mobility of our subjects and their distribution among certain types of jobs. These cannot indicate the trends which we saw working in the careers of individual subjects, which made us think of them in three groups: as the stationary, the circulatory and (naturally the largest group) those whose careers could not justly be described as either. That such differences should exist is to be expected. We have no doubt that temperament plays a large part in whether a career is nearer the stationary or the circulatory end of the scale. What interested us was the variety of influences, of which temperament was only one, which had gone to the shaping of individual careers in all three groups.

We shall illustrate this by an account of a subject who held only one post since qualification. From an earlier life not outwardly eventful she entered the Course at the age of thirty, straight from her social science training. Behind this lay some years of experience in general social work. She told us at her interview that when she took her present post in a mental hospital she had not intended to stay more than a few years and at least twice got as far as applying for other posts. Gradually, however, she began to identify herself with the hospital and a sense of loyalty to her medical superintendent, whose humane attitude she appreciated, prevented her from resigning; it seemed very unlikely at that time that anyone would apply for her post. Not less significant is the fact that developments within the hospital gave variety to her work. It needs to be remembered, when one is tempted to regard anyone as 'stagnating' in her job, that professional experience is in some circumstances enlarged as much by staying in a post as by leaving it. Finally, the hospital was conveniently situated for carrying out a double family responsibility which extended over the greater part of her thirteen years' stay. We have little doubt that this degree of stationariness represents some important element of personality. But the other determining factors exist and we should go far astray if we ignored them.

Our second example represents a more common form of the stationary tendency; here there is some changing of jobs but complete fidelity to a particular type of work. This subject entered with the intention of working in a child guidance clinic. After holding her first post of this kind for four years, she moved to a second, leaving it after a short period for another clinic directed by the same psychiatrist, but representing, in its relation to the community and the problems with which it faced her, a marked contrast to the clinic she had left. Here, at the time of her interview, she had remained for seven years; for some years the supervision of students had given her the satisfaction of trying herself out in a new function without the necessity of seeking variety in new surroundings. We can think of other subjects whose 'stationariness' seems to represent more obviously a dislike of change; in one case this corresponds to an unsettled early life and a satisfying personal life at the present time.

The larger group, which we have called 'circulatory', represents a wide range of situations and tendencies. The careers of some of these subjects show a more or less conscious pursuit of professional experience. One, after twelve years' practice as a psychiatric social worker in several posts both with children and adults, remarked at the time of her interview that she considered that her training was now, in a sense, complete. In the post to which she had recently moved she at last felt free to build up something for herself. In other cases the motives for change were less consciously educational. In the career of one subject with varied experience the chief conscious driving force seems to have been a sense of obligation to use her capacity, warmth of feeling and unusual energy in the service of the community. Her whole career as she described it gave the impression of a persistent search, even though personal and professional circumstances had deflected it considerably at times. She was now making full use of her qualities, specialized training and experience in an administrative post outside psychiatric social work. In another career there were traces of a recurrent urge to establish a new post and a tendency to pass on when this was accomplished, not because the essential interest of the first job had waned but in order to repeat the process. It seemed, too, that the coming of a psychiatric social worker colleague meant to her some loss of satisfaction.

Whatever underlying motives may have shaped them, none of these careers gives an impression of casualness, not even that of a subject who described herself as a 'born drifter'. 'Circumstances' rather than 'considerations', she declared, had shaped her career. It was not that she had held an unusual number of jobs but that, as she pointed out, there had been no planning. It is true that jobs came to her unsought, but, as far as one could judge, they came when she was obviously ready and fitted to take them.

In some instances, a professional purpose is not easy to trace. One of our subjects, talking of her own tendency to move from job to job, remarked that, if she were married and had a child, she might feel quite differently about her professional career. Other kinds of family obligations have affected many subjects' careers at certain periods. Such obligations can easily be viewed too negatively. It is interesting therefore to find a subject, whose own career has been moulded to a large extent, and for a time interrupted, by such obligations, asserting the positive importance of family background and family commitments for anyone engaged in psychiatric social work. Most of her work has been carried on where she has her roots, a fact which, in the eyes of her psychiatrist referee, has added much to its value.

In thinking over the material of our study we are struck by the apparently haphazard way in which the pieces in the field of employment seem to fall into place, and at the same time by the sense of something working itself out; some of the subjects were obviously impressed by this in their own careers. There were instances of apparent false starts, and of distress which might have been prevented if individuals had been given adequte information on which to reach their decisions. In some cases the value of unfortunate experiences was obvious to others and in some the subjects were also well aware of it. In the course of our study we asked a few whether they thought that more might have been done for them with regard to employment, either by the staff of the training course or by their professional association, which has indeed provided an appointments service from its early days. Of the few who thought that too little help had been given all had in mind the first post. A few considered that at the end of the training guidance might have been given about the general nature of the problems which students were likely to meet in different kinds of posts. A few felt that they might have been warned about difficulties of a personal kind generally known to exist in certain vacant posts. Yet one of them doubted, on looking back, whether she could have accepted advice before experiencing the difficulties for herself, and another, who had earlier felt that she should have been warned of the notorious difficulties of her first post, had become much less sure about this since she had herself taken part in the supervision of students.

The main theme of this chapter on professional careers is that of flux and of possibilities, some of them unforeseeable by any method of prediction. While we have dealt here more directly with training and practice, the question of selection has always been in the background. It is not only a matter of whether it should be possible at the stage of selection to distinguish between those whose vocational wanderings represent essential instability and those in whom they are purposive and may bring the subject happily to rest in psychiatric social work. It is the much wider question, as we have tried to show earlier, of how far it is possible, at a given point of time, to judge what a candidate will make of the experiences, both personal and professional, which are coming to her. Clearly what is needed is not so much improved techniques for detecting the presence in a candidate of particular qualities, as the development of skill in foreseeing a candidate's capacity for development through experiences of every kind, of which professional experiences form an important, though not necessarily the most important, part. More knowledge is needed of how careers do in fact work out. Studies along the lines indicated in this chapter might throw effective light upon some of the problems of selection, provided that they were intensive enough and also extensive, giving due weight to external circumstances and covering a subject's career before as well as after her specialized training. This has been beyond the scope of our study.

The tables given overleaf show the types of posts held by fifty of the subjects of the study and their mobility. They are presented as being of interest in relation to the discussion on careers in this and later chapters, but are not to be taken as a true sample.

Tables showing types of posts and mobility of fifty subjects over period from qualification (between 1934 to 1939 inclusive) to 1949.

TABLE I

FIRST POST AFTER QUALIFICATION

As psychiatric social worker				*Not as psychiatric social worker*		*Not in salaried post*
Clinical Children	Clinical Adults	Community care	Other	In social service	Other	
17	17	1	2	9	3	1

TABLE II

POST AT TIME OF STUDY

As psychiatric social worker				*Not as psychiatric social worker*		*Not in salaried post*
Clinical Children	Clinical Adults	Community care	Other	In social service	Other	
9	11	4	5	5	4	12*

* Includes eight who are caring for young families.

TABLE III

NUMBER OF SUBJECTS IN RELATION TO NUMBER OF POSTS HELD SINCE QUALIFICATION

(*a*)

All salaried posts

Number of Posts	1	2	3 or 4	5 or 6	7 and over
Number of subjects	3	8	18	15	6

(*b*)

Posts as psychiatric social workers

Number of Posts	1	2	3 or 4	5 or 6	7 and over
Number of subjects	10	10	17	12	1

Table IV

Number of Subjects in Relation to Number of *Types* of Posts Held Since Qualification

Categories used: (i) clinical (children)
(ii) clinical (adults)
(iii) community care
(iv) research and training
(v) other

Number of types of Posts	1	2	3	more than 3
Number of subjects	18	20	11	1

Note: The high number of those with experience of only one or two types is partly accounted for by the withdrawal of subjects early in their careers for the care of young families.

Table V

Number of Subjects Whose Period of Employment in any One Post Averaged:

Under 1 year	*1 year and up to 2 years*	*2 and up to 4 years*	*4 and up to 6 years*	*6 and up to 10 years*	*10 years and over*
6	13	22	4	3	2

CHAPTER VII

WORKING IN PARTNERSHIP

i

'How much do you use your psychiatric social worker?' As a question from one psychiatrist to another this seems at first hearing harmless enough, yet a psychiatrist who overheard the question among his medical colleagues found it 'indefensible and ethically improper'. If we tried it out on members of both professions, many in each might find it unobjectionable. It is a question nevertheless which serves as a good introduction to various problems which make themselves felt when psychiatrist and psychiatric social workers are working together.

There is something faintly shocking about the question when it is adapted and put into the mouth of a psychiatric social worker. Yet 'How much do you use your psychiatrist?' is not a quite inconceivable question to overhear where psychiatric social workers are talking at ease together. Perhaps the word 'use' in the second case would carry a hint of manipulation, a half humorous suggestion of getting one's own way without obtruding it. A psychiatrist once described the part of the psychiatric social worker in an adult out-patient clinic as that of 'mother' to the psychiatrist's 'father'. The 'mother' saw to it that the 'father' thought himself to be the head of his own household and that the household never forgot it. Both knew that it was she who, in not needing recognition, was really in charge of the situation, but this was never mentioned between them. We wonder how psychiatric social workers as a whole would regard the ethical propriety of so Victorian a view of both family and professional relationships. Yet it is not very different from a situation described by a psychiatric social worker, acting as referee for a colleague working in a child guidance clinic. She writes: 'I think the fact that Miss X can create a calm atmosphere in so hectically busy a clinic, can relinquish a good deal of her independence to Dr. Y, while having to put up with the inconveniences which result from the latter's arbitrariness, an indication of her psychiatric social work skill.'

In contrast to such subtleties, the question with which this chapter opens is presumably to be taken as a straightforward expression of the speaker's view, unconcealed and unexamined. The psychiatric social worker, it would seem to imply, is at his disposal to carry out his professional purposes. It is an attitude not hard to understand; we suspect too that the practice of some who might ask the question is better than their words. Nevertheless, a relationship is suggested which is incompatible with the responsible co-operation of a group of people, respecting each other's competence, who combine to apply their different training and experience to a common end. We shall return later to a suggestion, put forward by the psychiatrist who overheard the question, of how this kind of co-operation can be secured.

In the meantime it will be useful to examine, on the basis of our study, some of the relations in which psychiatrist and psychiatric social worker actually stand when working together, and how this influences the nature of the latter's job. We do not forget that the job goes on while the individuals concerned give place to others, and that this calls for constant readjustment. We sometimes notice a professional relationship between a particular psychiatrist and a particular psychiatric social worker, the success of which seems to depend so largely upon the working together of two unusual people that we wonder what the effect will be when one or other is replaced. The relatively permanent element is the structure or setting in which the co-operation takes place. This undoubtedly tends to promote a certain kind of professional relationship and it is for this reason that we propose to consider in succession the four main structures in which psychiatrist and psychiatric social worker are to be found working together, viz., child guidance clinics, mental hospitals, psychiatric out-patient clinics for adults and, lastly, community care.

ii

Burt has suggested that the real origin of the child guidance movement in this country is to be found in the Child Study Society, formed at the suggestion of Galton in 1893.[1] This might mean that child guidance is to be regarded simply as the recognition

[1] See p. 15 of *Autobiographical Sketch* quoted on p. 16.

of the emotional needs and difficulties of the individual child and the attempt to understand and meet them.[1] This is not the way in which the term 'child guidance' is used in this book. We are using it here in the commonly accepted sense of a professional method, by which the special knowledge and skill of different disciplines are brought to bear upon the problems of the individual child. In a child guidance clinic, where medicine, psychology and social work, in the persons of psychiatrist, clinical psychologist[2] and psychiatric social worker, are all intent upon a common aim, the scene for relationship is set. As we shall see when we pass on to the mental hospital, the recent origin of the child guidance method has an important bearing upon the place which the psychiatric social worker normally takes in the team. Compared with a worker in a mental hospital, she can be described as having been in at the start and as having a share in the forming of the traditions of the movement. In theory at least her special contribution is accepted as on a level with that of psychiatrist or psychologist in the regular case conferences characteristic of the child guidance clinic, where an ease of consultation is to be looked for only rarely achieved in any other setting in which a psychiatric social worker is likely to work. We must not, however, expect to find in the child guidance service of every local authority the conditions and attitudes which have developed in a well-established demonstration and training clinic, or overlook the special features of certain clinics forming part of hospital organizations where a different tradition survives.

As we considered the accounts of child guidance clinics which came to us in the course of our study from both psychiatrists and social workers, we thought that we saw them ranged between the poles of what we may perhaps dare to call the 'extraverted' and the 'introverted' types. As an example of the former we have an account of a busy clinic in which the psychiatrist takes an active part in the day-to-day administration. It is very much in touch with the world outside and furthers popular education in mental health through talks and discussions. In this the psychiatric social

[1] In Burt's scheme for a child guidance clinic (*Young Delinquent*, Univ. of London Press, Appendix II, pp. 617–27, 1925) an important place is given to social workers.

[2] We do not overlook the importance of the relationship between psychologist and psychiatric social worker, especially in child guidance. But this chapter is founded to a great extent upon the material of our study which, unfortunately, threw only a fitful light upon this subject.

worker, whose part in the organization of the clinic itself is restricted, takes her full share. If time allowed, the psychiatrist would like to see her getting in touch with local doctors, not only to advise them about the kind of cases to be referred to the clinic but also to discuss with them cases in their practice involving problems of family relationships. Although in this clinic consultation between psychiatrist and social worker is said to be frequent, there are no regular case conferences, the usual focus of the clinic team. Such a clinic must make for a different kind of relationship between members of the team from that of a clinic of the 'introverted' kind.

In one of these which was described to us, both the directing psychiatrist and social worker were inclined to reduce 'public relations' to a minimum, concentrating upon intensive case-work. Staff case conferences, as was to be expected, were held regularly. Perhaps the most notable contrast with the 'extraverted' clinic just described, where the psychiatric social worker is thought of rather as relating clinic to community than of exercising her function of relationship within the clinic itself, lies in the fact that in this clinic her counterpart is described as holding the clinic itself together, responsible for its atmosphere and playing the rôle of clinic 'mother'. Here psychiatric social worker and psychiatrist work in close relationship. The psychiatrist spoke of the need of the two to know each other very well indeed so that the meaning of each should be plain to the other. In another clinic of the same type, the psychiatrist expressed a doubt whether the Mental Health Course prepared students adequately to understand what the psychiatrist was doing and so to be able to co-operate with him through her own work with parents. In such clinics, the emphasis is not so much on frequent consultations over individual cases as on a fundamental understanding of what the other's part in the case really is. Such a relation implies mutual respect between professions.

We are not directly concerned here with the nature of the psychiatric social worker's share in a case; nevertheless the psychiatrist's views about this are likely to influence the relation between the two. One psychiatrist referee expressed his doubts about whether the psychiatric social worker was the right person to carry out the treatment of mothers, which he regarded as work for trained analysts, if these were available. The psychiatric social worker, in his view, would be better occupied in 'psychiatric *social* work' rather than therapy, which she was doing *faute de mieux*.

Exactly how the term 'psychiatric *social* work' was used here was not made clear, but such a view would seem to relegate the worker to the outskirts of the team and to imply that, however much her own contribution was appreciated, she would stand in a comparatively detached relation to the psychiatrist.

We need not assume that such a relation would necessarily make the job unsatisfactory to all social workers. An harmonious relation among those working to a common end is obviously desirable and, when two people are working on what is so intimately one problem as that represented by the mother and child who come to a child guidance clinic, lack of harmony between them is likely to be damaging. It is at the point of intensive treatment that their professional relationship is put to the severest test. At the same time a clinic is always more than the sum of its case-work, and the pattern of relationship in the clinic staff wider than that between psychiatrist and psychiatric social worker alone. In the clinic where the service is more diagnostic and advisory, a more general understanding among all the clinic team of each other's functions and a sense of common purpose could be enough to provide adequate conditions for psychiatric social work of a certain type. These indeed may be more congenial to some workers than the conditions of a clinic concentrating upon more intensive work. Even within the category of child guidance there is room for the expression of wide individual differences, and a worker who would be at ease at one end of the extraverted-introverted scale of clinics might well be most uneasy at the other.

If, as of course may happen, a psychiatric social worker passes from a child guidance clinic to a mental hospital, she will be struck by the contrast in conditions of work, and not least in the different relation in which she stands to the medical staff. A medical superintendent of a mental hospital, who in some ways had drawn his own worker into the life of the hospital to an unusual degree, was deploring the small number of newly trained psychiatric social workers who were ready to take up employment in mental hospitals. He had to admit, however, that, in contrast to the situation in other clinical posts open to them, in the mental hospital they would inevitably be somewhat 'extraneous'. The obviously medical nature of adult psychiatry and the history of the mental hospital service with its long tradition, into which the psychiatric social worker made a comparatively late entry, go far to account for this. She does not fit into the existing hierarchy;

even the question 'With whom shall the psychiatric social worker take her meals?' may, in a mental hospital, present quite serious difficulties!

This does not make for comfort, yet it ought to be remembered that this 'extraneousness' is part of a freedom which she herself values, the freedom to keep one foot in the hospital and one in the outer world, admittedly an uneasy stance. It is hard to see how it can be given up without loss of an essential part of her contribution to the hospital. We have suggested earlier that she represents one aspect of that opening outwards of the mental hospitals which was a comparatively late phase in their long history. Even by those who have wished for her appointment she may be felt as an enigmatic figure. If, as has sometimes happened, she has been imposed by a local authority upon a reluctant medical superintendent, her position may long remain a very difficult one. Even when her welcome at the hospital is genuinely warm, she may find that no one there knows what her functions are, or, a still more difficult position, that a pattern has been laid down for her within which she cannot make the contribution for which she believes her experience and training have fitted her. Usually she will discover some member of the staff who understands how her specialized service may be used, but she will have to accept the fact that missionary work within the hospital will continue to be called for even when the service seems to have been well established.

For a young student, who has not found her feet in some kind of professional work before training, to pass straight after qualification to a post of single psychiatric social worker in one of the large mental hospitals, perhaps of 2,000 beds, can be a severe ordeal. The strangeness of the setting, the mistakes which she will make as a result of her lack of first-hand knowledge of the legal machinery and the etiquette of a mental hospital, quite apart from her very limited experience of mental illness itself, all these can easily lead to a shrinking and apologetic attitude or an attempt to assert herself through demands for conditions and status, which, while perhaps not unreasonable in themselves, may be inappropriately made and ill-timed. On the other hand, for the social worker, whether experienced or not, with essential wisdom and the right blend of self-respect and humility, the mental hospital offers a challenge which has often been admirably taken up. To listen to accounts of psychiatric social work in mental hospitals is to listen to a story which soon begins to have a familiar ring. A period of more or less patient waiting, with experiences so discouraging that to resign might have seemed fully justified, is followed by the discovery of one or more members of the medical staff with whom it is possible to enter into a satisfactory professional relationship. Often this seems to arise out of a psychiatrist's sudden understanding of what psychiatric social work has meant in a single case. Opportunities open up and the worker, who may up to now have been employed more or less indiscriminately in obtaining social histories on all newly admitted patients, or in reporting on home conditions when the patient's discharge is being considered, now finds herself faced with a varied, if not always an informed, demand for her services. She now has to steer carefully between an over-rigid definition of her functions and a readiness to take on whatever she is asked to do. Someone who has worked through all this and, keeping her professional ideals, has established her place in the hospital, is a tempered blade indeed.

One of the subjects of our study described her experiences in a large mental hospital to which she went some eleven years ago, as soon as she had qualified. She was one of the older students of her year and impressed the training staff as being unusually mature, wise and sincere. As one would expect, she was able to tolerate an isolated job better than many, yet the situation even for her was bewildering enough. Unlike many newcomers to such a post she was not kept occupied by routine reports, and it was for her to decide where she could contribute most to the patients' welfare. She decided to devote most of her time to helping patients after their discharge to readjust to the world outside the hospital and, as she conceived it, this involved close personal work with both patients and relatives. No one in the hospital, as far as she could see, cared what she was doing. It is true that her own conviction that she was being of use to patients and their families would have justified her in her own eyes, 'even if the hospital had not known of her existence', yet the isolation in which she worked shook her professional confidence, so that she would sometimes wonder whether what she was doing was psychiatric social work at all. It was only when she left that she learned that the medical superintendent, who had recently come to the hospital, had noted and appreciated her work. It is not uncommon to find a psychiatric social worker in a mental hospital remarking that she would gladly exchange some of her freedom of action for what a worker in a child guidance clinic referred to as 'happy consultation' with the medical staff. Yet there are elements in work in a mental hospital which offer a specially congenial environment for some who might find the more intimate co-operation of a good child guidance clinic press upon them too closely.

In the course of our study we received an account from her medical superintendent of the work of a very able subject who had reached her first post in a mental hospital comparatively late in her career. We do not describe it as a typical situation, but as illustrating how the particular personalities of psychiatrist and psychiatric social worker may unite to determine the shape of the latter's job and their way of working together. After giving a list of duties so wide that it is hard to see where her speciality is conceived to lie, the medical superintendent adds: 'She seems willing to do anything which will promote the welfare of the patients or staff within the hospital or elsewhere.' That this lack of selectiveness has lowered the esteem in which she was held as a professional worker is ruled out by the tone of high appreciation with which the writer describes her intelligence, her competence and her 'excellent knowledge of her work'. He goes on to indicate the relationship between them. He finds her 'personally acceptable' and her intelligence and efficiency satisfying to work with. Yet he denies any knowledge of the motives which underlie her work: 'Whether she is naturally kindly, tolerant and understanding, or whether she has been schooled by her training to display these qualities, I do not know.' This presents a marked contrast to the kind of professional intimacy which the psychiatrist from a child guidance clinic, whom we have already quoted, thinks necessary for co-operation in case-work. The writer goes on to describe the subject as doing her work 'with the minimum of help and guidance from me. Unlike some psychiatric social workers of whom I have had experience, she is a person of few words. She does not encroach on my time by demanding lengthy discussions of her plans and detailed accounts of the work she has done. She often does things on her own initiative and the thing is done before I know anything about it, but I find that I invariably approve of her action.'

Since this described only the relations existing between the social worker and her medical superintendent, we add his comments on those with the rest of the medical staff. They are described as excellent. 'They have great respect for her and give her full credit for her efficiency. I think I am right in thinking that this appreciation of her ability is very little influenced by any positive emotional feelings for her as a person, but in her case I do not think that this makes co-operation with her by the medical staff any less effective.' The writer makes a point of adding that she calls forth warmth of feeling from patients and relatives.

It should be clear that we are not thinking of any stereotyped professional relationship belonging to a child guidance clinic or to a mental hospital; the importance of the personal element is obvious. Nevertheless we believe that conditions in a child guidance clinic and the nature of the work undertaken there conduce to the development of a closer professional relationship than in a mental hospital, where the psychiatric social worker's duties are likely to be carried out in greater detachment.

The psychiatric out-patient clinic for adults shows some of the characteristics of the child guidance clinic and of the mental hospital. Yet a psychiatrist whom we quoted earlier coupled it with the child guidance clinic as attracting newly trained workers away from the mental hospital, because here, as in child guidance, the psychiatric social worker is 'king pin number one'. It should be made clear that out-patient provision for adults is not all of one character. In the case of a department of psychological medicine of a general hospital the psychiatric social worker employed there will have deliberately chosen to work with adults in out-patient conditions. But it is common for a psychiatric social worker employed in a mental hospital to devote some of her time to out-patient clinics, staffed by the hospital though usually held elsewhere. We may assume that in accepting her post the worker will have chiefly in mind the conditions of work in the hospital itself, though the work which she will be called upon to do in the out-patient clinics may make the mental hospital post more attractive. In what follows we shall only distinguish between the two types of clinics where there seems special reason for doing so.

If the out-patient clinic for adults has an attraction which the mental hospital lacks, wherein does it lie? Not, we think, in any greater appreciation by the psychiatrist of what the social worker can do. The suggestion that in mental hospitals she must always remain more or less 'extraneous' would seem to come nearer the mark. The usual problems dealt with in a clinic for adults are, like those of a mental hospital, more essentially medical than those referred to a child guidance clinic. On the other hand, even when the clinic is part of the structure of the mental hospital, it might be regarded as that part of the hospital most in touch with the needs and ideas of the community which it serves, and perhaps also least bound by mental hospital tradition. Here the psychiatric social worker, by virtue of her training and experience as a social worker, can never be really extraneous. Here she might be expected to feel at home.

From accounts which have come to us it would seem that the exact part which she plays in an adult out-patient clinic varies considerably. In many cases she is not only responsible for planning the clinic session but for directly running it. How far she spends her time as receptionist will partly depend upon the nursing staff available. A psychiatric social worker on her first day of work at an adult out-patient clinic, where several psychiatrists interviewed patients screened off in one large room, on asking where the psychiatric social worker usually sat, was told, 'Miss X (her predecessor) never sat down.' We understand that this situation was quickly remedied and we should like to think that it was unique. In many clinics the psychiatric social worker gives most of her time to interviews with patients and relatives in a room of her own, yet we get the impression that it is rare for her to be able to give undivided attention to her own case-work. One pictures her as always to some extent conscious of the activities of the clinic, of the feelings of staff and clientèle and even of the unseen community outside, and concerned in a special sense about shortcomings in the running of the clinic, such as unsuitable quarters or unreasonable waiting for interviews.

There is no doubt that the variety of skill called for in such a clinic, the assurance of having an important function to perform there and the many contacts which it affords with general social problems and with other workers in the field of social welfare make work in an adult out-patient clinic satisfying to those of a certain temperament and outlook. Here, in the broadest sense, they may exercise their talent for relationship in which, according to a psychiatrist referee in charge of a large psychiatric out-patient clinic, they are 'first-rate'. In its own way the adult out-patient clinic might perhaps be thought of as demanding maternal qualities, but rather those of the old woman who lived in a shoe than those of the 'mother' of a child guidance clinic, in the sense of the psychiatrist quoted earlier. It would be understandable if these two kinds of clinics, however much their conditions differ, should attract away from mental hospitals some who might find satisfaction there in the nature of the work itself. Nevertheless, the figures quoted in Chapter II show that mental hospitals exercise their own attraction.

It would seem that conditions of work in an out-patient clinic for adults are often more favourable than those in a mental hospital for consultation between psychiatric social worker and psychiatrist in spite of the long, crowded sessions which characterize many; we sometimes hear of relations established at an out-patient clinic of a mental hospital leading to more satisfactory co-operation within the hospital. Yet it is not unusual to find the psychiatrist handing over to the psychiatric social worker cases which she is expected to 'carry' without referring them back to him unless some unforeseen feature reveals itself. When the worker is experienced and ready to take responsibility, has confidence in the psychiatrist's judgment in selecting the cases to refer to her in this way, and has moreover adequate time for case-work, a post at a psychiatric out-patient clinic can be a very satisfying one. Naturally it is rare for all these conditions to be fulfilled. One psychiatric social worker spoke to us of her work at an out-patient clinic of a mental hospital. She is an experienced worker and can 'say what she likes' at the clinic. Her own view is that if she is used as a 'social specialist' it is less because of her specialized training than because she has been some time at the hospital. She finds that psychiatrists tend to hand over neurotic patients to her entirely. If only for lack of time, she is unable to hold long interviews at the clinic and can attempt little more than environmental readjustment of a practical kind, such as help with work or recreation, while recognizing that these measures are often quite inadequate. She is disturbed when patients ask her when their 'treatment' is to begin, thus shouldering responsibility for shortcomings in the clinic which are largely beyond her control, a subject to which we shall return.

In this chapter we have drawn considerably upon the material of our special study. With regard to community service the changing situation makes this method less useful since our study referred exclusively to community service as provided by a voluntary body, whereas, at the time of writing, this service is chiefly carried out in the health departments of local authorities. In describing the development of psychiatric social work in Great Britain, we have given an account of the after-care scheme for ex-service psychiatric casualties and discussed in that connexion problems of the relations between psychiatrist and psychiatric social worker very relevant to the theme of this chapter. In later chapters we have considered in more general terms the position of the psychiatric social worker in the mental health service under the National Health Service Act. Here we shall only touch very briefly on a few of the special points involved in community care, whether under voluntary or statutory auspices.

The scene of community care is not a clinical one. It is the social scene in its broadest sense, in which the psychiatric social worker should feel at home by reason of her discipline as social worker. Her relation with the psychiatrist cannot be the same as in psychiatric clinic or mental hospital. It seems likely that she will always have to be prepared to make decisions in certain cases about whether a client should or should not be referred to a psychiatrist. Much of the time she will be applying her psychiatric-social knowledge and skill in situations and with individuals who, however disturbed, come within the range of normality. Her psychiatric training and experience should allow her to judge when a pathological condition demands expert help, which she is not competent to provide. This makes great demands on her judgment, and we have expressed the opinion elsewhere that this is no work for any but experienced and professionally mature people. We do not see how the needs of the situation can be met except by a very flexible kind of co-operation between psychiatrist and psychiatric social worker, and mutual trust. This is more easily secured if the latter is obviously competent as a social worker; on this basis her superimposed training and experience in psychiatric matters is much more likely to be taken seriously. A tranquil acceptance of the profession of her origin is perhaps the best guarantee that she will respect the profession of the psychiatrist, and recognize where her own professional boundaries lie.

iii

We have already referred, in writing of mental hospitals, to the difficulty which a psychiatric social worker is almost bound to meet of discovering where, in any particular hospital, she can play her part most usefully. This means striking a balance between what is expected of her and what she herself considers her functions to be. This is part of a general problem which is not confined to mental hospitals; it seems, however, to appear there in its most urgent form.

It is safe to assume that there is more work to be done to which her special training and experience could reasonably be applied than she will have time to undertake. Every case admitted to clinic or hospital has a social aspect; the proportion of cases in which she will play a part will depend on the amount of time available, and upon a judgment which has to be made about whether she shall intervene in a particular case. Who is to make this essentially social judgment? Can it be left to the psychiatrist? If not, should not the psychiatric social worker be brought into every case at the stage of diagnosis, when a decision is made about the line of treatment? The conditions of a child guidance clinic tend to make this the rule.

One of the psychiatrist referees from a mental hospital advocated a flexible kind of co-operation at this stage. He thought not only that psychiatrist and psychiatric social worker should decide together on which cases a social history was called for but also, if a history was needed, on which of the two should take it, since particular circumstances would make now one and now the other the more suitable. There is no need to underline the value of co-operation of this kind, but experienced social workers know how difficult it is to achieve in the work of a mental hospital as a whole. In a well staffed department of psychiatric social work the time of a senior worker would clearly be well spent upon whatever form of co-operative selection was appropriate to the conditions of the particular hospital. It is probable that equally good results are reached by methods which may appear very different. The medical superintendent of a large progressive mental hospital thought that a senior psychiatrist should be appointed to 'vet' the work undertaken by social workers, so that time should not be wasted on unsuitable cases referred by the less experienced members of the medical staff. From the context of the writer's suggestion it was clear that this did not imply any lack of appreciation of what psychiatric social workers have to give, but aimed to protect them from dissipating it. The 'vetting' would presumably take place in consultation with them. The view is often expressed by those who work in mental hospitals, especially those who work there single-handed, that, although they are more than fully occupied, they cannot be sure that they are not missing some of those cases to which they could contribute most. Perhaps this will always be true to some extent. Yet even a few starting points of good co-operation are ground for encouragement and the psychiatric social worker, if she is willing to feel her way, may suddenly find that the work she is doing does not come to her in as haphazard a way as she had imagined and that a process of selection has been taking place which, however imperfect, is yet suited to that particular place and time.

We may approach the same subject by another route. One of us remembers being present at a series of instructive discussions among psychiatric social workers of a certain hospital, meeting under the chairmanship of a psychiatrist. The subject most under discussion at the time was that of the hospital's out-patient clinics. These were suffering from an almost complete lack of secretarial and administrative help, so that the psychiatric social worker attached to the clinics felt herself constantly diverted from her special functions to act as receptionist and clerk. The psychiatrist replied to her very natural protests by asking why she took upon herself this wide responsibility for the running of the clinics? To all of us with experience of clinics of this kind the question seemed exasperatingly unpractical. An undirected clinic would be likely to mean that patients waited even longer than at present to see the psychiatrist, and would certainly tend to cause a general disquiet among all those who attended it. The work of the psychiatrist himself would certainly not remain unaffected. There would be repercussions outside which might result in the clinic's losing the confidence of the community which it was set up to serve. The suggestion that the psychiatric social worker, if she felt that she, like the psychiatrist, had specialized work to do, should simply insist on doing it and detach herself from all general responsibility for the clinic's teaming life, seemed almost monstrous. It was only later, in colder blood, that one saw that the question, impractical as it might seem, probed deep into the psychiatric social worker's conception of herself.

A psychiatrist at an out-patient clinic would be likely to take it for granted that the psychiatric social worker should undertake this general responsibility. The fundamental question is, however, whether it is not really she who is the cause of his doing so, because in fact the running of the clinic seems to her to be as much her real work as her more specialized work with individuals. Even if a clinic were provided with the best possible administrative help, would she not still feel a general responsibility? If so, is this the result of an over-developed conscience or a wish to manage and dominate, or can we find a more respectable explanation? When we discussed this with an experienced psychiatric social worker who had recently taken up work in a large and busy clinic, and so was still viewing it with undimmed eyes, she told us that, even with the best administrative help, she would certainly still remain tuned in to the various personal encounters and exchanges which make up the clinic's life. This confirms the general impression we have gained.

This is not unconnected with a proposition put to the psychiatric social workers by the psychiatrist at the same discussion which, to judge by the strength with which they always reacted, touched some quite profound feeling among them. Why, asked the psychiatrist, could the social worker not be content with what in effect was the honourable position of a social specialist, leaving it to the psychiatrist to refer to her such cases as, in his opinion, called for her specialized skill? As he saw it, her position was comparable to that of the pathologist to whom a case would be referred for an opinion based on his specialized knowledge, which the psychiatrist himself would never claim to have. In the same way the psychiatric social worker would be called in to a case for a limited purpose, and when that was fulfilled, would, like the pathologist, make her exit. It was interesting to find that this group of workers, holding a variety of views about the nature of their work, rose as a body against this comparison with the pathological laboratory whenever it was suggested.

Unfortunately urgent practical problems prevented at the time any fruitful discussion of why they felt so deeply and positively that the comparison did not fit their case. We do not think that they were specially concerned about their position. The psychiatrist himself thought that he was urging upon them a position far more honourable than that in which, in their failure to stick to their last, they seemed determined to place themselves. It might be that in the comparison with the pathologist they sensed an over-emphasis upon the scientific and technical which was at variance with their own conception of their work. We are more inclined to think that what brought from these assembled psychiatric social workers something like a cry of protest was that the comparison did indeed seem to make them 'extraneous'. It excluded them from the kind of co-operation with the psychiatrist which they regarded as essential to their best work. Perhaps the psychiatric social worker is asking to have things both ways. The fact that, as a social worker, her base is historically in the community keeps the door out of the hospital or clinic open to her; she can never be completely absorbed into it and this is a situation she values. Yet she does not want to be pushed even so far as the circumference of clinical work into however splendid an isolation. She feels her need to develop in the closest relation with psychiatry, to learn from it continuously, and in regard to any particular case, to work in a partnership with the psychiatrist which does justice to the wholeness of the patient, who is an individual belonging to a social environment.

In our special study we asked no direct question about the relationship between psychiatrist and psychiatric social worker, yet the subject arose indirectly. Our first impression was that psychiatric social workers were, on the whole, more critical of psychiatrists than psychiatrists were of them. If it is true that the relationship between them is more important to the worker in the carrying out of her own work, and, one may perhaps add, more a subject of conscious thought, this is what we should expect. It must be borne in mind, however, that our study also gives much evidence of psychiatric social workers' appreciation of psychiatrists with whom they work and the genuine co-operation which has existed between them, especially when that association has been of long standing. This is easily left unmentioned, whereas the frictions and irritations which may arise in the course of trying to establish good working relations with psychiatrists in the making more often reach expression.

Criticisms of psychiatrists are usually concerned with two things: first, slowness to apply their psychiatric understanding and skill to those persons who form the patient's human environment; second, failure to understand what psychiatric social workers have been trained to undertake, and the difficulty they have in admitting her to genuine professional responsibility in cases in which she is called upon to exercise her special functions. It is the second which concerns us here. A psychiatric social worker of good judgment was looking back over many years of work in a mental hospital. She commented on the difficult situation which sometimes arose in accepting the leadership of psychiatrists still in training, who had seen so much less of mental illness than she. This made a false and embarrassing position when, as sometimes happened, they seemed unable to allow her responsibility in cases in which her help had been called in on the social side. This reminds us of incidents in training when an intelligent student who, on entering, was already an experienced social worker, would be working on a case with a doctor who was in process of training in psychiatry. When, as sometimes happened, the latter would adopt a somewhat authoritative attitude, the student would not unnaturally be resentful, since she recognized his limitations both in psychiatry and in the province in which she herself was expert. What complicated the situation was that, while recognizing this intellectually, in her own capacity of student and perhaps also of psychiatric social worker, she wanted a psychiatrist, even a potential one, to be all-knowing and all-wise and found it difficult to admit to herself how widely psychiatrists in fact differ in these respects. We have the general impression that the psychiatric social worker looks for a strong lead from the psychiatrist with whom she works, and expects to learn from him. It was said to us of a particularly able psychiatric social worker that she went about looking for a 'maestro'. Perhaps the tendency is not uncommon among us and our critical attitude may be explained as that of the disappointed idealist who has set up for others an unattainable standard.

Psychiatric social workers are fortunate in that psychiatrists have not placed them in this particular false position. It is true that various expectations have been aroused about them, through the selectiveness of their training course and perhaps also through their portentous title, yet, as a rule, the psychiatric social worker has to prove her worth to the psychiatrist as an individual, just as in case-work she has to work without the support of the traditional prestige on which the doctor can draw. Examining the opinions of psychiatric social workers expressed by the psychiatrists who acted as referees in our special study, we find material interesting enough to be given in some detail. Of the forty-two psychiatrist referees who were prepared to rate the work of their subjects on a three-point scale, thirty-two gave an A, nine a B, and one a C rating. This was unexpected and we looked round for an explanation. We wondered whether the referees had found it difficult, when it came to something as definite as a rating, to give anything but a favourable verdict, but in fact we found that the high ratings were well supported by the comments which accompanied them. Turning back to training records and comparing the psychiatrists' ratings with the standard of work reached at that stage, we found that twenty-one out of the thirty-two rated A by psychiatrist referees had also been regarded as of A quality during training.

Thus only eleven raised a problem. Of some of these it was suggested during training that they would not reveal their real quality as long as they remained in the position of students. In the case of others it is easy to see in retrospect that in favourable conditions, of which the most important might well be a good relationship with the right psychiatrist, they would do valuable work. Perhaps, after all, the ratings were not as surprising as they had seemed at first sight. Nevertheless, we were still impressed by their generosity and reminded ourselves that some of the referees might have been influenced by their knowledge that we ourselves had a considerable responsibility for the training of the subjects whom they were assessing.

There were, however, other facts which might, we thought, have a bearing on the question of generous ratings. In the few cases where the psychiatrists' ratings suggested that the promise of training had not been fulfilled, none of the subjects had been working with her referee for more than five years. As against this, there were many among those rated A who had worked with their referees for six or seven years and some for considerably longer, up to thirteen years. It is reasonable to see a connexion between the higher ratings and the greater opportunity for the growth of understanding and for mutual adjustment which these long periods of collaboration afford. Another fact emerged from our study, for which we could adduce parallels from our general experience. A number of psychiatrist referees, while expressing the greatest appreciation of the subjects whose work they were assessing, referred darkly to other psychiatric social workers whom they had met or heard of, about whose fitness for the profession they could have told a very different tale. We can only guess at what this means. Perhaps the psychiatrist becomes to some extent identified with the social worker with whom he is working at the time. In any case it is presumably difficult for him to see in the ordinary, and we hope capable, person with whom he works from day to day, the rather strange being which her not altogether fortunate title is apt to conjure up. The psychiatrist's esteem for a psychiatric social worker would seem to grow through working with her, and if this conclusion is too flattering, perhaps we may be allowed to hold it provisionally, to offset some unflattering criticisms which we have to report in a later chapter.

We have already considered the question of the medical direction of psychiatric social work in the conditions of community service. The fact of medical direction seems to be so generally accepted in clinical settings, particularly in the more unequivocally medical settings of work with adults, that the subject was rarely mentioned in the course of our study. How the direction was applied naturally gave rise to more discussion. On this subject we should like to give an extract from a memorandum by the psychiatrist referee to whom we referred at the opening of this chapter, from which we have leave to quote. After enumerating certain functions of a clinic team which are vested in the psychiatrist alone as a 'duly qualified medical practitioner', the writer points out that this places him in a peculiar relation to all patients attending the clinic. He goes on, however, to make recommendations for dealing with 'responsibility' within the team:

> 'That responsibility for the care and treatment of patients shall be vested in the team with the psychiatrist continuing to assume responsibility for those functions which by law he alone can fulfil. This places upon the psychiatrist the responsibility not only of his specific function but that of permitting to his colleagues full therapeutic autonomy, while being prepared at any moment to assume the full responsibility for the conduct of any case.
>
> 'There is therefore an obligation upon each member of the team to make truly known to the others the course and progress of cases in their care. . . . The degree to which this is possible in any one team is probably the measure of the security and maturity of the individual members of that team.'

While we believe that this liberal interpretation of the way a clinic team can work together closely represents what is happening in some child guidance clinics, it will make members of other clinic teams compare this ideal rather wistfully with the reality they know. The last sentence quoted deserves attention. Professional maturity is sometimes of slow growth and it would be unwise to assume that every qualified psychiatric social worker is necessarily ready for or would welcome the exacting combination of liberty and close association here implied.

A letter came to us in the course of our study putting a point of view about medical direction which may be unconsciously influencing some of those who, after a considerable period of time in clinic or hospital, leave psychiatric social work to apply their training and experience outside the clinical field. It should be noted that the writer's longest and most recent experience has been in a child guidance clinic where the relationship within the team was, we believe, much like that recommended in the memorandum just quoted. After referring to the inferior pay and conditions of work of psychiatric social workers as compared with those of other members of the team, she goes on to say: 'I think that in any profession there should always be the possibility of reaching the top even if only for a very few. That a very experienced first-rate psychiatric social worker's work should always depend on the psychiatrist, whether experienced or inexperienced, seems to me to lead to a sense of insecurity within the profession, although, of course, there are many teams where such factors are of no importance. In ideal conditions—which are very rare—I think a psychiatric social worker's work in a child guidance clinic is entirely satisfying.' We have quoted this passage not because we want to question the necessity of medical direction in child guidance, but to illustrate an attitude of mind which must be taken into account in predicting the future of psychiatric social work.

We recall two referees, both of whose subjects were persons of unusual intelligence and energy, suggesting that psychiatric social work might not hold them much longer. As we indicate later[1] we by no means necessarily regard as 'wastage' in any depreciatory sense the passing of psychiatric social workers beyond the borders of 'social work undertaken in relation with psychiatry'. It is important however to understand what is happening and to distinguish between 'wastage' which is a sign of healthy growth and 'wastage' which points to dissatisfaction within the profession. In any honest exploration of the second, we should expect many of the issues raised in this chapter to claim attention.

[1] See Chapter IX, iii.

CHAPTER VIII

SERVICE IN CLINICS AND HOSPITALS

i

With the case studies of Chapter III in mind we shall now consider what it is that psychiatric social workers do in clinics and hospitals within the conditions which we have tried to indicate in Chapter VII. Work in community care is left for later discussion, except in so far as it shares the common features of all psychiatric social work. We recognize that work with children and work with adults have their special problems in spite of their common aim; in this chapter we shall treat these two branches separately or together as seems most natural and convenient.

We shall try first to state what we regard as fundamental to psychiatric social work. Some will see it as essentially a statement of social case-work itself. We think of psychiatric social work at its simplest as an endeavour to help individuals, in personal difficulties as social beings, to reach a better understanding of the baffling and frustrating situations in which they are placed and to release in themselves unsuspected capacities for dealing with them. Since the field of the psychiatric social worker is mental illness and maladjustments of personality and personal relations, the difficulties in which she offers her services are likely to involve a high degree of emotional disturbance, whether the individual with whom she works is the patient himself or someone in his environment. Because of her psychiatric training this will be her special concern, even when in the course of her work she has to take into account many problems of a practical kind which will be familiar to her as a social worker. How far she attempts to deal with these herself will depend upon a number of circumstances and upon her own choice; where these are available she will commonly enlist the help of appropriate specialized services. Her dual training will not allow her to see individual and social, material and personal, in isolation. The most practical problems, such as the shortage of houses, will present themselves to her fraught with emotional implications for individuals.

It has sometimes been stressed, and rightly, that the process of helping someone in personal difficulties is one and indivisible. Yet while they cannot be distinguished in time, there are always two processes at work. In one information is assembled and an attempt made to understand it. In the other, an attempt is made to build upon the basis of knowledge, and something which we may provisionally call treatment is undertaken. While the first process calls for specific facts and for logical thinking, the second is more in the nature of an art and demands from the worker a high degree of intuition and a disciplined use of her personality. Yet each process is constantly reinforcing the other. The distinction is indeed an abstract one and the qualities called for in the practice of an art are nowhere more needed than in the opening phase, when the diagnostic aim may be uppermost.

In attempting to present so briefly what the psychiatric social worker does, we may have given an impression of someone actively grappling with the client's problems. What she in fact undertakes is quite different. We may think of her as someone who, while she is in a position to see aspects of the client's situation which are hidden from him, will not assume that she knows in advance what is good for him or that it would help fundamentally in the solution of his difficulties if he were persuaded to see things from her standpoint. On the contrary, she sees him as someone whose need is not only to perceive the cause of his immediate difficulties but to understand himself as the person who has come to be involved in them, and, above all, to discover in himself a source of fuller living, within which the difficulties, in so far as they remain, will take on a different character. She will see her own rôle as one of giving courage for the adventure, not through persuasion and externally applied reassurance, but through the building up of a relationship between herself and the client within which he will feel confident and free enough to make his own discoveries. As a warmly interested yet disinterested and uncriticizing person, the worker can be relied upon for support when self-discovery means the stirring up of troubled waters. She will recognize that in any such relation a phase of dependence or hostility on the part of the client must be accepted as a natural element in what is taking place between them. How far she will help him to understand his experience, including his relationship with herself, and how far she will stand back and allow things to work themselves out with little intervention will depend upon the particular worker and the particular client. There is room within this general method for work of many kinds and at many levels.

We have described a way of approach which some social workers will always have followed, led by their natural gift for dealing with people and by their intuitive grasp of a particular client's need. What we have in mind differs in being deliberately adopted on the basis of recent discoveries about the development of personality and the significance of human relationships and behaviour, and is capable of cultivation and to some extent communicable. The essential features of this way of service are brought out more clearly if it is compared with another way of helping individuals, which has a long and honourable history, and will, we may be sure, continue to play its part in social work. The worker who follows this other path usually attempts to influence the client on the basis of reason, even when her work is founded upon a warm relationship, in which the client will often play a dependent rôle. The distinguishing mark of this approach is that the worker ,from a fixed point of conviction, believes that she knows what the client needs and sees further than he does. Her aim is to get him to stand where she does and see his problem from her own supposed point of vantage. Such an approach can be made crudely and dictatorially, but there is no reason to think of it in its caricatured form. The strength of the worker's convictions and the overt nature of the persuasion used meet the needs of certain people where more tentative methods may fail.

Of these two ways of helping someone in personal difficulties, the first is the psychiatric social worker's chosen method and is in keeping with what she has learned through her specialized training and experience. She believes that such enlightenment as results from it will lead to interior changes more likely to be lasting in their effect than those resulting from any kind of external pressure. Within the relationship built up between worker and client there is a place, however, for many elements, among them some to which we have referred under the second method, including the worker's own basis of conviction and the use of reasoning. There is a sense in which the method characteristic of psychiatric social work can be called 'passive', in its receptiveness of what the client has to say and its acceptance of his right to make his own discoveries and to use what she has to offer in his own way or to reject it. But it is sometimes implied that the worker should be 'passive' in relation to the client in a sense which seems to leave her too unsubstantial to afford support to anyone in distress of mind. The richer and more developed the inner life of the worker, the more she will have to give in her relation with the client. That she has reached or is moving towards some unified attitude to life does not imply imposing this upon those she tries to help. Unless, however, she can represent in herself the possibilities of integration and order, it is hard to see how the client can find in her the security which he needs.[1]

In an earlier chapter we noted how difficult the subjects of our study found it to distinguish between personal and professional elements in their development as persons engaged in professional work. We do not find the abstraction of a professional self very useful in our own thinking. It is what the worker is as a complete person that is brought into play in the course of personal service and behind this lies her whole personal development up to that time. This does not imply an amateurish conception of her work. If, as we believe, she enters into a relation with a client as a whole person, it is all the more necessary that she should aim at the fullest possible understanding of herself as well as of what happens between her and the client, since, at the beginning at least, it is she who must take responsibility for the relationship between them.

It is sometimes suggested that the psychiatric social worker should never give advice. Such a view would seem to imply that her position approximates to that of the psycho-analyst, working within the strict conditions of his highly specialized task and free to select carefully the patients whom he treats. Since we are now trying to describe what is common to the whole range of psychiatric social work, this analogy is misleading. There seems, moreover, to be some confusion of thought about the term 'advice'. The main function of a Citizens' Advice Bureau is to allow a client to make a decision on the basis of sound knowledge. That among its clients

[1] A Discussion Group on training for social work at the British Conference on Social Work in 1948 decided that 'universities must exercise great tolerance in rejecting social work students on any other grounds than intellectual', but that while 'moral unorthodoxy should not lead to rejection . . . moral incoherence, that is the possession of no consistent moral standard, could be ground for rejection.' *Outlook for Social Work*, National Council for Social Service, 1949, p. 32 (not obtainable).

are those who need help of a different kind does not concern us here. In psychiatric social work there is a place for advice of this nature, based upon knowledge derived by the worker from her professional training and experience, which the client has not been in a position to acquire. In itself it involves no more than allowing him to make an informed rather than an ignorant choice or decision.

One may take the case of the psychiatric social worker attached to a mental hospital who keeps in touch with the family of a patient after he has left hospital. The psychiatrist will presumably have explained to the relative, as far as the latter is able to understand, the nature of the patient's illness and, when this applies, the symptoms and changes in personality which are to be expected. But the worker, seeing the patient at home or at least hearing of what happens as patient and family are in daily process of readjusting to each other, will be able to apply and supplement the general information given by the psychiatrist, which is apt to have little meaning for the relatives until difficulties actually arise. She will speak with some authority, not because she believes she could herself deal with the situation better (indeed she will often be humbled at the thought of how inadequate she herself would be in the relative's place) but because she has a wider, if more shallow, experience of mental illness, and opportunities of drawing upon expert knowledge which the relative cannot have, and also because she is not personally involved. This enables her to translate what the psychiatrist has said into more concrete and individual terms. Because, however, she also understands the emotional relationship which is likely to develop between herself and the relative, she will realize that what she offers is never mere information. Other elements will enter, such as the authority of the hospital which she represents and her personal influence with the relative. She will thus consider the giving of advice as part of the whole complex process of service and will not be blind to its dangers.

The position of a worker engaged in a child guidance clinic offers a parallel. It is questionable whether a psychiatric social worker should concern herself immediately with the mother's present difficulties in dealing with her child's behaviour. That the mother will ask for advice is natural, but an experienced worker will know that the meaning of such a request will depend on many things and she will often withhold it.[1] Nevertheless, she would be a

[1] See Case I of Chapter III, p. 41.

very doctrinaire worker who would refuse in all circumstances to impart to the mother, in a form which she could use, the results of accumulated knowledge about child behaviour. In some cases to give such advice, or rather information, would be futile; in other cases again it might be harmful in that it would deceptively allay anxiety which needed to be given free vent. The decision to give or withhold advice of this informative kind must rest upon the worker's understanding of the whole process of the mother's attempt at self-discovery within her relationship with the worker at a particular point of time.

Up to now we have been thinking of the client as someone who is capable of self-direction, but psychiatric social work, by its very nature, involves dealing with some individuals who, temporarily or, as far as one can foretell, permanently, have not this capacity or only to a very small degree. Taking the profession as a whole, the psychiatric social worker is not justified in refusing; because she has a preferred method, to deal with those to whom the method is not appropriate, or in forcing the client into the method's Procrustean bed. It may be necessary with a depressed patient for the burden of decision in some social or personal matter to be temporarily lifted from his shoulders; disregard of this fact might even involve a risk of suicide.

In some cases the individual will be able to resume full self-direction in the course of time, but in others the problem is presented in a more lasting form. This may be met in the person of the actual patient or of a relative, faced, in the patient, with a task beyond his powers. The need here may be for long sustained support and, although in the present shortage of specialized workers there may be strong reason for delegating such work, the psychiatric social worker cannot refuse responsibility for such cases. In accepting it she will be showing the trained worker's appreciation of the infinite variety of individual needs at all levels of mental health, and will be doing no violence to her belief in self-direction for everyone capable of exercising it. To impose freedom upon someone who is not able to use it can be an insidious and particularly dangerous form of tyranny.

The passing of the National Health Service Act of 1946 faced psychiatric social workers with a possibility which, although its actual effects have been limited, disturbed them considerably at the time. It was suggested that they should be included among those to be appointed, in succession to relieving officers, as duly authorized officers with duties under the Lunacy and Mental Treatment Acts. Of the various arguments put forward for and against such an innovation, it was evidently those concerned with the use of compulsion which were most deeply felt. The main issue was whether this was inconsistent with the principles of psychiatric social work or whether, in spite of the practical difficulties involved, the new function should be accepted, since to repudiate it would be not only to make a doubtfully justifiable claim for exemption from a distasteful duty, but also to miss an opportunity of applying the essential principles of psychiatric social work in conditions which would test them to the utmost. Such work might be taken as representing the far end of the scale at the other end of which stands the process of self-discovery, freely undertaken by the client within a relationship established with the worker. We would suggest that it should be possible for the essential contribution of psychiatric social work to be made over the whole extent of this scale, though not by each individual worker to the same degree.

Students not unnaturally emerge from their year of specialized training with very different ideas of what it is that they have now become. Many would accept the phrase 'social workers with psychiatric understanding' as a just description, while others would hardly recognize themselves in such a guise. This is not surprising in view of the variety of experience in general social work which students bring with them to the Course. One may have held a responsible post as social worker for many years before the idea of training as a psychiatric social worker occurred to her, while another may have undertaken a social science training with only such practical experience in social work as was demanded of her, entirely in order to qualify for it. We should expect the feeling of these two towards social work and social workers to be worlds apart. Yet the fidelity of psychiatric social workers to their original calling seems to depend to a great extent on more personal factors. With some what they are now doing seems to have developed naturally out of social work, but for others it is more in the nature of an escape and may bear the marks of protest against being associated with something from which they have tried to move away. The direction in which they are drawn is naturally that of psychiatry; in some cases the fundamental attraction would seem to be that of medicine as a whole, and in others that of psychotherapy.

'Home visiting' is a topic which illustrates a certain confusion of thought related to this situation. It is associated in the public mind with the idea of social workers and it is true that this has been one of their characteristic ways of carrying out their work. The term itself conveys only the fact that the meeting between client and social worker takes place in the client's domain, not in a clinic or hospital or in the office of an agency. In the course of any one case, interviews may take place now in the office, now in the home, according to the kind of work which has at the moment to be done. The term covers interviews of various kinds; at one end of the scale is the visit of frank inspection, at the other what is often called 'friendly visiting', of old and infirm or merely lonely people. 'Home visiting' has come to be associated on the one hand with unwarrantable intrusion and on the other with a rather formless relationship between social worker and client, which, it is felt, should have no place in professional case-work.

Home visiting in psychiatric social work has been more characteristic of work with adults than of child guidance, partly, but not wholly, as a result of conditions of work. There seems, however, to be a growing tendency for workers in mental hospitals to depend more than formerly upon interviews conducted at hospital or at out-patient clinic. In child guidance an interview at the clinic is certainly the normal medium for psychiatric social work, though there is considerable variety from clinic to clinic in the use which is made of the additional method of home visiting. Several of those who contributed to our study told how, after the emphasis laid during their child guidance training on the clinic interview, they were surprised to find that, when the conditions in which they worked, such as a wide county service, made this necessary, interviews both for taking social histories and treatment could be carried out successfully in the home.

Home visiting undoubtedly calls for much consideration in relation to psychiatric social work, if only because its essential character seems to have become confused with other issues. One of the psychiatric referees deplored the fact that psychiatric social workers were less ready than formerly to visit the patient's home. In his view to pay a good home visit called for much greater skill than taking a history in a hospital or clinic. One clue to this reluctance is perhaps given in a statement of one of the subjects of our study, working in a newly established child guidance clinic. She laid stress upon the importance of insisting on clinic interviews, because of the tendency in her clinic to regard her simply as a social worker and to expect her to spend most of her time visiting. This may well have been wise policy in these particular circumstances, but it does not touch the central question. The wish to dissociate themselves from the tradition of social work seems to us to enter quite often into discussions among psychiatric social workers about the relative value of home visits and clinic interviews, making it difficult for them to consider the matter on its merits. And with the reaction from the traditional methods of social work there would seem to be a positive attraction to the methods of other members of the clinic team, notably of the psychiatrist. It is very understandable. The psychiatrist, interviewing in clinic or hospital, is professionally protected in a way that the psychiatric social worker, at large in the community, can never be. Her position, between institution and community, can be a source of considerable strain, and it is tempting to abandon it for a position more secure and defined. Perhaps too the idea of a clinic interview unwittingly represents for the psychiatric social worker something of the psychiatrist's prestige.

We do not wish to enter here into a discussion of the value of home visiting. The arguments for the hospital or clinic interview are weighty. Yet we believe that any further restriction of home visiting might mean impoverishment for the psychiatric social worker herself and so for the client. What we want to emphasize here is that it is important for the profession that it should build up its methods, not as a result of revulsion from or attraction to anything at all, but according to its own essential character and needs.

ii

While the assembling and interpreting of facts is a process which can be distinguished from the process which follows as a result of it, in any one case the two cannot in fact be separated. With this reminder, we shall go on to consider the 'social history' and the various problems which it raises in psychiatric social work. We have become so used to the term that we may not often give much thought to the meaning of the word 'social' in this context. It might mean one of three things or the three combined: a history taken by a social worker, a history taken not from a patient but from someone in his social environment, or a history which emphasizes the importance of social experiences, irrespective of who takes the history or gives the information. Here, combining all three senses, we shall take a social history to mean an account of the patient composed by a social worker on the basis of the information given by someone closely associated with him and familiar with his social environment, which gives special attention to environmental influences, including such elements as family relationships from early days onwards, material conditions such as economic level and stability, and the cultural influences of racial, religious, occupational and other groups.

The psychiatric social worker in a clinical post may reach, as a result of her own investigation, a 'social diagnosis'. By her selection of material for her social history and the way she presents it she cannot altogether avoid suggesting the inferences she has drawn, even if she does not deliberately try to interpret her findings. But her history is a contribution to a 'combined operation', and without the findings of psychiatrist, and, especially in the case of children, of psychologist, her inferences can only be partial and may be misleading. This is something which a student of psychiatric social work often has to learn by repeated experience, especially perhaps in work with adults. She has also to remember that, although material may have to be organized and presented at a particular point of time, the 'social history' is ideally something which is unfolding itself throughout the whole process of a case.

The use made of the social history in different types of work differs considerably; we shall distinguish here child guidance clinic, mental hospital and out-patient clinic for adults, and observation ward. In the child guidance clinic, because the conditions dealt with are, as a rule, of a less medical kind, less emphasis tends to be placed on diagnosis. The social history is regarded mainly as the social worker's contribution to the attempt of a clinic team to reach a general assessment of the child's needs and decide how and through whom they can best be met. In some clinics a considerable proportion of the social worker's time may be spent upon cases which, as far as she is concerned, end at this stage. Yet since the assumption is that the social worker who takes the social history from the mother of the child patient may later be working with her in treatment, it is generally accepted that the social worker may have to forgo information which it is desirable to have, if to seek it at an early stage might impede the building up of a good relation between the mother and herself.

In work with adults, where the medical element figures more largely, the part played by the social history is somewhat different.

In the early days of psychiatric social work in this country workers in mental hospitals found that the taking of such histories was, of all their functions, the one most easily accepted by psychiatrists. The danger was lest they should come to be regarded primarily as history takers.[1] It was a nice point how far and how long they should leave unquestioned the psychiatrist's view of their main function, while trying to demonstrate their usefulness in other directions. It could not be assumed in work with adults that interviews for the taking of the social history would be recognized by the medical staff as laying the foundation of a relationship between informant and social worker on which social treatment might later be built. It was for the psychiatric social worker herself to get this point of view understood and this she could not hope to do unless she herself genuinely accepted the importance in the diagnosis of mental illness of accurate detailed information. It has occasionally been necessary for her in the past to make a stand against the suggestion that not only should the social history be presented according to a broad scheme 'kept under the blotter', but that it should be taken down at an interview in the form of answers to a set of stereotyped questions. This has been generally resisted, not only because it was felt to prevent the free development of a relationship between client and worker, but because it was held to be a method which, except with information of the most formal kind, did not in fact lead to the accuracy desired. A circumstantial story told in the speaker's own way and in his own order, with the minimum of guidance from the worker, is likely to be more reliable and more economical, in that such facts as appear are given as part of the fabric of life and carry with them a kind of unpremeditated commentary.

Some psychiatric social workers have been anxious, not without reason, lest their social histories should be misused, especially when circulated among psychiatrists with some of whom they would not be in direct contact. They themselves would regard a social history as one aspect of a patient's story, the point of view of someone not necessarily more immune than the patient himself from mental distortion and bias. If, however, the patient were so seriously mentally disturbed at the time the history was taken that he could not give an account of himself, this could easily come to be regarded as the authorized version of his story, and its relative nature for-

[1] 'Historians' has been used as the title of some of the workers in a mental hospital in U.S.A.

gotten. It is important to remain aware of the responsible nature of social history taking. When this becomes a routine, such awareness is easily blunted.

We notice a change in the demand for social histories. At least in those mental hospitals where psychiatric social workers have been established for some time and have demonstrated the value of their work in social treatment, the demand has become more discriminating. One of us engaged in the supervision of students of the Mental Health Course, in a hospital active in the training of psychiatrists, found herself after the war in the unfamiliar position of having to stimulate artificially a demand for social histories, in order to provide her own students with this indispensable discipline. What made this especially interesting was that there was no lack of demand for psychiatric social work in other directions. This notable reversal of the situation contains a useful challenge to psychiatric social workers to review what they have been doing. The social history which they have taken in the past has, in fact, tended to cover much the same ground as the history taken from the patient by the psychiatrist; this is not necessarily the best use of her special training and experience. Psychiatric social workers in earlier days were apt to complain that, in taking the social history, they were being used to 'save the psychiatrist's time'. This was not, perhaps, a reason for great distress; there is, however, something wrong when she is regarded as primarily a time saver. This is indeed only likely to occur if she limits her social history to a narrowly factual account of what she thinks the psychiatrist wants to know. A social history taken by a psychiatric social worker who is fully alive to the social implications of what is told her makes demands upon the psychiatrist, in bringing home to him the complexity of the patient's social situation and his effect upon his environment. It is not unknown for a psychiatrist to express this by pushing away the knowledge which the psychiatric social worker brings to him because, once accepted, it would involve for him, if not action which he is not prepared to take, at least a wider range of thinking about the patient and his needs.[1]

The social history of the psychiatric social worker in an observation ward presents essentially the same problems as the social

[1] We are reminded of a story of a medical superintendent of a mental hospital to which a psychiatric social worker had recently been appointed in the early days of the profession, who said to her, when she reported that an ex-patient was again apparently becoming homicidal, 'You mustn't *tell* me things like that or I shall have to do something about it.'

history in clinic or hospital, but throws them into higher relief. In the observation ward it undoubtedly takes precedence for the social worker over any other kind of duty. Here the two purposes of history-taking, to supply accurate information for diagnosis, often particularly important in these cases, and to establish a relationship with the informant as a basis of future work, are especially clearly marked. The limit imposed by law on the length of time a patient may remain in the observation ward gives urgency to the whole procedure. As a rule the history has to be based upon a single interview, often with a person who has just been through a period of extreme stress, and may be labouring under a feeling of guilt over his part in the patient's loss of liberty. It is exceptional for the social worker in the observation ward to be herself responsible for sustained social work on the case. This is likely to be in the hands of her counterpart attached to mental hospital or out-patient clinic. What the worker at the observation ward is trying to establish is not a relationship which she herself will later be able to develop, but one which prepares for the entry into the case of some other worker, whose way of working may differ a good deal from her own. The relative when seen at the observation ward will often make use of the opportunity to talk with less than usual reserve. A worker who tried to stem such confidences would miss a unique opportunity to help, yet she herself will not be able to watch for the reaction which so often occurs when a reticent person, to her own surprise, has given vent to emotion. It seems to us that the qualities needed for this work are sometimes underestimated.

Up to this point we have been considering the social history taken from a relative. There are occasions, particularly in community service, where the psychiatric social worker may be dealing with someone who comes to her for help without having been in touch with a psychiatrist, and with whom, moreover, it would be quite inappropriate to raise the question of obtaining a history through any other person. She will sometimes need to learn direct from him enough of his history to allow her to decide if and how she can help him. In such a case she will be under no obligation at this stage to supply another with diagnostic material, and her pace will be set entirely by the needs of the case as she herself is dealing with it. The history will be a 'social history' only by virtue of her trained sensitiveness to the importance of social experiences and the client's response to it in telling his story.

The situation is different when, as sometimes happens in an adult out-patient clinic, the psychiatric social worker, on her own initiative, or at the express wish of the psychiatrist, takes a history from a patient himself before the psychiatrist sees him. We know that in a very busy out-patient clinic this arrangement may be the best that can be made in the circumstances, but we suggest that a psychiatric social worker should consider carefully, first, whether she should undertake the function at all, and second, if she decides to do so, how she can carry it out, not as an imitation of the work usually done by a psychiatrist, but in a way that is consistent with the special character of her service. Unwisely handled the taking of a preliminary history from a patient in advance of the first psychiatric interview may well confuse the patient and take the edge off this interview. We are not sure that the worker is justified in accepting the situation only because the psychiatrist himself sees nothing wrong in it. To subject a patient to two interviews in quick succession at his first attendance at a clinic is to ask much of him in emotional adjustment. It seems to us one of the psychiatric social worker's obligations to remain aware of the importance of matters of this kind.

iii

If we say that a psychiatric social worker has a part to play in the treatment of psychiatric cases, we believe that we shall meet with general agreement. It is a different matter if we suggest applying the word 'treatment' to the actual part she plays. We seem to remember that in the early days psychiatric social workers in this country tended to use the term 'treatment' for what they were doing, but used it, as it were, behind closed doors. We can illustrate the fear which this reflects from our own study, from the case of an experienced worker of whom her psychiatrist referee wrote in the highest terms. In the schedule which aimed at discovering how she felt about undertaking the various duties which her job comprised, she wrote of what we were bold enough to call 'treatment interviews with relatives': 'Enjoyed them thoroughly during training at the child guidance clinic—in a job always felt very inadequate and terrified of encroaching on psychiatrist's preserves', adding characteristically: 'Looking back I know that a number of my interviews had a therapeutic value but more because some of the patients and relatives liked and trusted me than because of anything that could really be called treatment.'

We hope that time has done a good deal to allay anxiety and that a mutual understanding is developing, which will make the use of the word 'preserves' out of place. Among psychiatrists, however, the psychiatric social worker's part in a case is often referred to as 'social adjustment'. This term would probably be accepted by most psychiatric social workers as describing part of what they do, at least in certain cases. It has however picked up some unfortunate associations and easily suggests to her that relegation to the circumference of a case which we discussed in an earlier chapter. The term 'social adjustment' should have a double meaning, implying both an attempt to adjust environment, human and otherwise, to the patient, where his personal limitations seem to make this necessary, and also an attempt to help the patient to deal with his environment, at times actively and at times in the sense of being reconciled to it in its imperfections. Too often, however, it is limited to the first of these meanings and used to imply 'social manipulation' in its narrowest sense[1], such as urging upon a local authority a patient's claims for priority in housing. Such a step is often an entirely appropriate part of psychiatric social work; it is only when it is undertaken in a fragmentary way, not as something arising out of the needs of the case as a whole, that it may be neither truly psychiatric nor truly social.

The medical use of the word treatment is only one of a wide range of meanings, within which there is surely room for what the psychiatric social worker does. It therefore seems permissible to use this word in preference to 'adjustment' when we need a single term to describe the whole of her contribution to the combined management of a case, rather than her contribution to diagnosis.

It is not easy, as we found in our study, to be sure at what level any particular psychiatric social worker is working. This is partly a matter of terminology. Experience teaches that one must not always take an impressive description of what is being done at its face value; work of high quality, on the other hand, may be pre-

[1] While two of the psychiatrist referees of our study evidently regarded skill in manipulation as worthy of praise, when a psychiatric social worker referee spoke of her colleague as a 'manipulator', the implications were evidently different. An interesting discussion of 'manipulation', used in a very positive sense, occurs in *Psychiatric Principles in Casework* by Grete L. Bibring, where she writes: 'Manipulation offers in many ways a new experience to the patient which may have a more or less lasting influence on him in the same way that similar experience in life may result in changed attitudes in a positive or negative sense.' Kasius, Cora (ed.): *Principles and Techniques in Social Casework*, Family Service Association of America, 1950, p. 379.

sented by the doer in a very modest guise. An experienced worker, intelligent and self-critical, whose work we believe to be anything but superficial, told us how she tended to feel bewildered and cast down when she listened to other psychiatric social workers talking of what they were doing. Then one day, in the course of conversation with a colleague, her own work on a case was handed back to her, clothed in the terminology which had so impressed and confused her. Was this really what she had been doing? If so she had some measure by which to assess the achievements of her colleagues, which no longer seemed quite so impressive.

There are, however, real differences between what one worker and another are actually doing in treatment. Some of the differences are dependent upon the branch of work concerned, some upon the way of working characteristic of particular clinics or hospitals, others again upon the individual's conception of her functions, and her capacity. We shall need to distinguish between child guidance and work where the patient is an adult, and shall turn first to work in a child guidance clinic.

The characteristic work of a psychiatric social worker in such a clinic is illustrated by the first case study in Chapter III, which shows the ground being prepared for sustained work between the clinic worker and the mother of a child referred to the clinic as a patient. We shall confine ourselves here to this characteristic rôle, since it is distinguished most clearly, though not absolutely, from the part played by the worker where the patient is an adult. It should have become clear, however, in Chapter VII that even in the most 'introverted' clinic the duties of the social worker comprise more than her individual case-work. We would add that in the case-work itself, fathers as well as mothers may be the subjects of social treatment, though it is easy to understand why work with mothers takes first place. This is a matter which varies considerably from clinic to clinic.

Among the many different kinds of work with mothers carried out by the psychiatric social worker in child guidance clinics, we may distinguish two. There is, first, work in which the emphasis is placed upon the child's problem. However widely the work may range it is always tethered to this. In the second type of treatment the work with the mother takes on a life of its own, though the case remains under the general direction of the psychiatrist. The only limits set to the treatment of the mother in such cases are her own needs as an individual, the extent to which she is prepared to pursue the treatment with the worker and the latter's belief in her own capacity to undertake it. The position of such a mother, once she starts treatment, is not essentially different from that of someone who has, in the first instance, sought help on her own account. In practice, of course, the two types of treatment are not so clearly distinguished as this. No work with the mother of a child patient is likely to be effective unless she is led to recognize the relations between the child's problems and her own, and to accept help on her own account. This point is well illustrated in the first case study. Some workers will bring it into the open at an early stage, while others will allow the mother to reach an understanding of the position at her own pace, sometimes leaving it implicit between them to the end.

It is important to remember that both kinds of work take place within the conditions of a clinic team. The kind and amount of consultation between psychiatrist and psychiatric social worker will depend to some extent on the nature of the work each undertakes. When work with the mother remains closely related to the problems of the child, one would expect that the two would need to consult frequently about the progress of the case; when this does not happen, it would seem to be due to the exigencies of an overbusy clinic. In the second type of treatment there would often appear to be a different kind of co-operation. In some instances, at least, the psychiatrist believes the psychiatric social worker to be capable of work beyond the capacity of many of her colleagues. It may then be assumed that psychiatrist and worker have reached a mutual understanding of how each thinks and works, so that consultation on individual cases is called for less frequently. We do not think that those working in this way form a large group. It may be assumed that most of them have undergone a personal analysis and some will have received special help from the psychiatrist with whom they are working. The Mental Health Course, as several subjects pointed out, was a door which led them to these later experiences. It is important that this should be understood, since for a course of one year, of wide and varied content, to pretend to train its students to undertake something approximating to lay analysis would rightly bring it into disrepute.

It would seem to be at this point, before we pass over to work with adults, that we might usefully stop to examine what distinguishes the work undertaken by psychiatric social workers from that of psychiatrists when both are trying to help individuals by psychological means. We recognize, of course, the variety which exists in the psychotherapy practised by the psychiatrist with whom psychistric social workers are associated, ranging from that of the qualified psychoanalyst adapting his methods to the conditions of clinic and hospital to the more empirical therapy of those whose work is based upon their general psychiatric training and experience. For our present purpose we shall discount the differences on both sides.

First, it has to be remembered that the psychiatrist has behind him the prestige and authority of his profession. This may not be an unmixed advantage since, while it often leads to the quick establishment of trust, it may also arouse an expectation of wonder-working which can be an embarrassment. Psychiatric social work, while it may share some of the general prestige of hospital or clinic, has yet a lay element which makes for freedom in relations with those it serves.

Secondly, we would return to our tentative suggestion that the psychiatric social worker's psychistric understanding is superimposed upon an understanding of the 'body-social' comparable to the psychiatrist's understanding of the human organism by virtue of his medical training. The consequence is that each, in a treatment interview, will be especially attuned to catch the meaning of half-expressed communications and signs of quite different kinds. Indeed their different set of interest is likely to draw from the person with whom they are dealing behaviour and communications which are also unwittingly different. Moreover, it seems likely that the psychiatric social worker will be the more constantly aware of the two that the weekly hour of treatment, crucial as it may be, forms a very small part of the mother's whole span of experience, where innumerable external influences play upon and impede or encourage development. She will remember that the interior drama played out between mother and child, which she is helping the mother to bring out of the depths into clearer consciousness, is also an exterior drama, played out against such concrete things as cramped accommodation or inadequate housekeeping allowance. Perhaps she may sometimes wish that it were otherwise, but for anyone who has come to see things as a social worker this kind of awareness seems inescapable.

Our third point is not unconnected with the second. In her constant concern with the patient as a member of society, her range of attention is, and in our view should be, wider than the psychiatrist's. While for both the focus of the case will always be the patient, for her the people by whom the patient is affected and whom he affects take on a reality involving not only obligations towards the patient, but needs and rights of their own which she cannot ignore. It is not uncommon for a psychiatric social worker to be critical of a psychiatrist's handling of relatives. In this she may be failing to allow for the limitations which are inherent in the concentration upon the patient to which the psychiatrist is committed. The moral seems to be that the work of the two is complementary in a very real sense. We would not wish the differences to be abolished but rather that they should on both sides be more fully understood.

Fourthly, it might be thought that a distinction could be drawn between the work of psychiatrist and psychiatric social worker on the lines that the former is concerned with both the conscious and the unconscious processes of the mind, while the latter confines herself to the conscious processes or material on the point of becoming conscious. Yet this criterion presents difficulties. We have assumed throughout that when she reaches the end of the Mental Health Course a student will have gained some understanding of the theories of unconscious processes and how these make themselves felt in individual behaviour and personal relations. This understanding becomes increasingly real to her through case-work before and after qualification. It should lie behind all her work, and without it any attempts to help individuals by psychological means would be unthinkable. One of the psychiatrist referees suggested that staleness was likely to creep into the job of a psychiatric social worker unless her work was somehow related to her inner life; this would depend upon her maintaining an interest in the unconscious side of the emotional life of the people she dealt with, 'not just paddling on the surface'. It will be noted that the emphasis here is on 'interest' and that it is not suggested that psychiatric social workers as a whole should undertake work of an analytic kind. We have already tried to make our position in this matter clear. Nevertheless, it would seem that the distinction conscious-unconscious does not afford a useful criterion for our present purpose.

We would mention one further difference. The person whom the psychiatrist treats is always someone who is referred for, or himself seeks, psychiatric help as patient—a sick person. The position of the psychiatric social worker is less clear-cut.[1] As the third case study illustrates, she may indeed be working with the patient, the mentally sick or disturbed person who forms the centre of a case. But her work in child guidance, as well as much of her work with adults, will be with someone in the patient's environment. Subjects of our study slipped often into the use of the term 'patient' for the mother of a child patient in a child guidance clinic. This is easily understandable and perhaps harmless. In the second type of treatment of mothers discussed the term is indeed not inappropriate. Nevertheless, we would suggest that it is better avoided. While it is essential for progress that the mother in a child guidance case should feel her own involvement in the child's problem, yet, even when seriously in need of help through psychological means, she may remain well within the generally accepted limits of mental health.

There are, however, cases in which the psychiatric social worker, in the course of her work with individuals in the patient's environment, will discover that she is working with someone who should, in his own right, be a patient in the fullest technical sense. It may be that the condition is of long standing but up to now has been concealed, or it may be that the work done with the psychiatric social worker has brought to light more serious problems. This has to be faced. If the social worker, instead of working constantly, as she does, in association with psychiatry, were working in isolation, such a serious possibility would cast suspicion upon her work as a whole. We would take it rather as confirmation of the need for close and continuous co-operation between psychiatrist and psychiatric social worker, so that the latter, as soon as she becomes uneasy about the mental condition of an individual with whom she is working, naturally calls in the psychiatrist's aid. The training of the Mental Health Course should have taught her to recognize such a situation at an early stage, and to understand the limits of her competence.

iv

Work with adults usually involves a wider range of duties, though not necessarily of problems, than is to be found in an

[1] In making this comparison we are not forgetting those who, when they seek the help of an analyst, have a more positive aim and neither feel themselves as sick people nor are regarded in this way by others. These do not come within the range of psychiatric social work.

average child guidance clinic, if only because the worker with adults is habitually associated both with patients and relatives, while it is not usual for the social worker in a child guidance team to have more than a general and passing contact with the child patient.[1] Moreover the worker with adults is apt to be concerned with a greater proportion of general social work, even if she delegates its actual performance, than is usual with clinic workers.

Taking as the most characteristic feature of work with adults the fact that the worker often maintains direct contact with the patient, we shall consider first some of the points raised by the third of the case studies, where contact with relatives plays almost no part. It might be objected in the case of Agnes Gifford that the relations between patient and worker were left too undefined and some of the methods used were unprofessional. It is worth considering these criticisms in their bearing upon the varying conditions which determine in a paticular case of work with adults what rôle the worker shall play. The pattern is not laid down for her in advance as clearly as in a child guidance clinic. In this particular case it is of the greatest importance that, during the first phase, the patient was undergoing regular psychotherapy, so that her relation with the psychiatrist was quite clearly defined. Moreover, she herself was an intuitive person, quick to grasp a situation and to adapt herself to it. The psychiatric social work might have needed very different handling if the patient had been seeing the psychiatrist only occasionally or if work on the case had been left entirely with the social worker. It might also have been handled quite differently if patient and worker had been different kinds of people. In every case it is the responsibility of the psychiatric social worker to understand what she is doing. In our view great flexibility is permissible and even demanded in direct work with the patients, and it is always a matter of individual judgment how much will be made explicit. The apparently unprofessional steps in the case we have described, such as the unconventional setting of the interviews and the giving of the worker's private telephone number, must be viewed in this light. They were the result of professional judgment on individual circumstances which may, of course, have been either well or ill advised.

The interweaving between inner and outer reality is unusually

[1] In certain clinics psychiatric social workers, by special arrangement, undertake some direct individual work with children.

clear in this case, as is the psychiatric social worker's part in the whole. Treatment causes disturbance of behaviour of a kind to be felt within the patient's working environment and the worker intervenes to help those concerned to understand, and so to tolerate such behaviour more easily while the phase lasts. Or fantasy (in this case about her mother), coming to the surface in treatment, calls for action on the plane of outer reality. For the psychiatrist in such a case to step out of one kind of reality into another might be harmful to treatment. The psychiatric social worker, in touch with the psychiatrist but with her feet in the community where the testing of the fantasy has to take place, can intervene without any prejudice to her rôle; indeed it is just this threading of one's way between inner and outer which is characteristic of it.

In this case contact with the patient has been kept over a period of some sixteen years, but at very different degrees of intensity. For the greater part of the time the approach has been made spontaneously and at varying intervals by the patient herself, and there has been nothing which could technically be called 'after-care'. By quite a natural process the conditions imposed and accepted as part of a professional relationship have eventually dissolved, and two people, who once stood to each other in the relationship of psychiatric social worker and patient, now meet as two human beings, with different experiences and ideas, which they enjoy sharing. Naturally, the old relationship is contained in the present one, but forms no more serious barrier than the fact that two congenial people have once stood to each other in the relation of teacher and taught. This potential friendship is surely present wherever two people come together in a process of professional service.

When we turn to those cases in which psychiatric social work is undertaken chiefly with some person in the patient's environment, we have something to compare with the work with mothers carried out in a child guidance clinic. Yet the fact that the patient is an adult, at least in years, influences the whole nature of the work. This is true even when there enters into the case such a problem as the patient's release from a dominating mother, so familiar to child guidance clinics. This problem is vividly illustrated in the second case study, though here the severity of the mother's own mental derangement makes the case atypical, though by no means without parallel in the experience of many workers. The adult patient's attitude towards the psychiatric social worker's establishing a relation with someone in his environment is itself a problem which does not arise in at all the same degree in the case of a child patient, though it may with an adolescent. Nevertheless, most psychiatric social workers with adults will remember cases in which such work has in fact proved possible. Out of the large case-load which seems especially to be the lot of workers with adults will emerge some cases in which a sustained relationship develops, by means of which a process of self-discovery and release is supported and encouraged. The conditions imposed by the special nature of each case have to be accepted, and a judgment reached about where in a patient's environment, if at all, psychiatric social 'treatment' can be applied.

In work with adults the 'relative' may be a parent or son or daughter, husband or wife, or someone else in a comparable position in regard to the patient. Psychiatric social workers, we believe, vary considerably in their readiness to undertake sustained work with the partner of a patient when the problem is mainly a marital one, although they will expect to meet many such cases in the general couse of their work. The training of the Mental Health Course should have made them more able to understand the factors underlying marital problems, but will also have made them more aware of their extreme complexity. Age and personal and professional experience outside training are likely to influence their practice in this matter.

Working as she does in adult cases, now with the patient and now with relatives, the psychiatric social worker will have to consider whether it is possible for her to maintain any but a very light contact with more than one of them at one time. A typically difficult situation is the discharge to his home of a patient with whom the psychiatric social worker has maintained a relationship during his stay in hospital concurrently with a relationship with a member of his home environment. To maintain at the same time a relationship with the patient, a mentally ill person in hospital, and with the relative who remains behind in the environment which the patient has left, will always need judicious handling, but the difference in the nature and setting of the relationships is usually enough to keep the situation reasonably clear. When however the patient takes his place again as husband or son or brother of the relative with whom the worker, in his absence, has built up a relationship, founded in the first place upon his illness, the situation can easily become seriously confused. A change in the balance of relationships may be necessary and perhaps a lightening of both.

The psychiatric social worker will sometimes complain that psychiatrists tend to refer to her the 'psychopath' or the 'hopeless neurotic', either when direct psychiatric treatment has been tried and failed or when it is not available. Sometimes she has grounds for complaining about the way in which her help has been called in and may suspect that the psychiatrist has no clear idea of what her part in the case might be. Having reached the end of his resources, and perhaps his patience, he still does not like to leave the patient in the void. But the referal may be a reasonable one nevertheless. Moreover, there are many psychiatrists who call in the worker's help with due consultation and with good understanding of the scope and limitations of what may be expected of her in cases such as these. We ourselves believe that the psychiatric social worker's position and characteristic way of working make it possible for her to contribute something to these cases, which can be effective, even if it be within narrow limits, where formal psychiatry has apparently failed.

We shall take by way of illustration someone whom a crisis, one in what seems an inevitable series, has brought within the field of psychiatry. The superficial picture is of a person who seems, in some curious way, bent upon his own ruin, one who seems to have only a rudimentary sense of belonging to the community and who causes social disturbances wherever he goes. Because his motives are so deeply overlaid, he is apt to give rise to a sense of mysterious confusion in those who come within his orbit.

There are several reasons why the psychiatric social worker may be able to bring a steadying influence into the situation. Like the psychiatrist she will realize that any progress in social adjustment can only be made within the limits of the patient's handicaps of personality. This should at least save her from joining in the chorus of exasperation which is apt to accompany such a patient on his way. Sometimes, moreover, he is able to make direct use of her help (often fitfully and perhaps only at long intervals), all the more easily because of her rather undefined position in comparison with the psychiatrist's, who cannot divest himself of his medical authority. At the same time, while he can expect from the psychiatric social worker an understanding of his difficulty as a social misfit, she represents, as a social worker, that affirmation of an individual's obligation towards society which is present in the patient to some degree, and for which he often seems half glad to find support.

The course of such a patient as we have described may continue to present a series of major or minor disasters and it may be that little can be done to help him directly. The responsibility of the psychiatric social worker does not, however, end with the patient. She is concerned no less with the effect of the patient on his environment and here her scope is wide indeed. Into the turmoil which is the natural result of his attitudes and behaviour, it is her part to bring some understanding of his disability and of its expression in a-social and even anti-social behaviour. Some of its sting may be removed if it is no longer felt as a personal or social affront. If those who suffer through the patient's behaviour can be helped to accept him without an over-anxious sense of responsibility for his actions, tension may be lowered and the patient himself may reap an indirect benefit. Experience seems to support this, yet no psychiatric social worker can feel complacent about what she may hope to effect in cases such as these; the terms 'success' or 'failure' are here particularly difficult to apply.

It has been suggested that the psychiatric social worker tends to be an optimist when compared with the psychiatrist. Does this mean that she is less ready to look facts in the face? Or is it that she expects less and so is pleased with results which would leave a psychiatrist unsatisfied? Or is her experience in her own field of a more encouraging kind than his? Whatever the answer to the first two questions we believe that the answer to the third is 'yes'. However imaginatively the psychiatrist may fill in his patient's background, the latter is still someone seen in a clinic or hospital. The social worker, on the other hand, should be able to see him always in relation to the social group from which he has come, so that his experience in hospital or clinic, however prolonged, is felt by her as no more than an episode in a life history which is interwoven with the whole development of the community to which he belongs. And on the whole the point from which she views the scene is the more conducive to optimism. The psychiatrist is ready to make allowances for individual differences in his assessment of mental health. But the social worker is constantly reminded to make allowances for differences of behaviour between social groups, and to recognize that these may all come within the limits of social health. There are certain people who, as patients or relatives, are dubbed 'stupid' by the hospital staff. It is not uncommon to find a social worker resenting this on their behalf. She has seen them in their natural surroundings, in social groups, where unconscious adjustments have resulted in a workable relation between individual and environment making for social competence within narrow limits. A patient with a residue of symptoms after severe mental illness can sometimes be carried in such a family group with far less strain on those around him than the hospital had dared to hope when he was discharged, and may even make unexpected progress. Such a group is not necessarily socially acceptable by any theoretical standards, but this is where the patient is at home and where he can find the tolerance and stimulus which he needs.

Naturally it is not always in his original environment that a patient will show himself at this unanticipated best, but the psychiatric social worker cannot escape the conviction that for every person with mental disabilities there exists, if only it could be found, a social setting in which he would go beyond his supposed capacity for living. E. L. Thomas describes a war-time experiment in which a group of seriously unstable people were temporarily absorbed, with the guidance of a psychiatric social worker, into a rural community. She writes of the powers of quite ordinary people when challenged, provided that they are given some support, to deal with really difficult problems at close quarters and adds, 'I am repeatedly struck by the fact that people, including patients, so frequently transcend their apparent handicaps and limitations, and it seems to me that this reserve of energy, which can be released in time of crisis, is of very special interest to the psychiatric social worker'.[1] It is the contemplation of experiences like this that gives the psychiatric social worker a tempered optimism, not founded on any statistics of success and failure. The social scene itself presents a spontaneity and natural interplay which is missing in the inevitably artificial conditions of hospital or clinic. A worker of long experience will always be on the alert for unforeseen combinations of circumstances, including the development in a patient's life of a new personal relationship, which will transform the situation. This is the state of mind in which, in the face of countless disappointments, optimism is able to survive.

[1] Thomas, E. L.: 'The Rôle of the Psychiatric Social Worker', *British Journal of Psychiatric Social Work*, 4, 1950, p. 24.

CHAPTER IX

SERVICE IN WIDER FIELDS

i

We implied in the last chapter that psychiatric social workers feel a special kind of responsibility for the impact of the service in which they are employed upon the community which it is planned to serve. The director of a child guidance clinic or the medical superintendent of a mental hospital is naturally very much concerned with the same question, and carries the responsibility at the level of policy. The psychologist in a clinic will be in touch with an important but limited section of public opinion, should the general liaison between clinic and schools be in his hands. But the social worker, even if she works in the most 'introverted clinic', is likely to be kept continuously aware of how the service which she represents is regarded, both among those working in the field of social welfare and among ordinary citizens who may have occasion to use it. This is especially true if she does not resist the pull of her own case-work outwards into the community.

It is often said that she has a particular responsibility for interpretation, not in the special analytic meaning of the term but in the sense of bringing about a greater understanding between those whose lack of familiarity with each other's language and ways of thinking keeps them more or less apart. This responsibility applies not only to a patient's relatives but to the 'man in the street', with whom her work brings her professionally into more frequent contact than the psychiatrist's, and with whom, as a less highly specialized professional person, she herself has more in common. When she is tempted, as she often is, to envy the more demonstrable expertness of colleagues of other disciplines, she may remind herself that all specialization carries with it its own disqualifications. The advantage of the limitations of her own specialized knowledge is brought home to her when, as may occasionally happen, she listens to some highly trained psychiatrist interviewing a patient or relative and recognizes the gulf formed by the psychiatrist's expert knowledge and the other's ignorance of his particular field, a gulf which only a high degree of imagination on the part of the psychiatrist is able to bridge. In contrast, the psychiatric social worker, with her absence of medical training, is never so remote from the ignorance of those to whom she is trying to interpret some psychiatric situation that she cannot sense their unformulated questions.

Other aspects of her interpretive function are mentioned by two referees, both tutors in university departments of social science. One of them, whose subject is employed in a child guidance clinic, writes of her as having a kind of consultant rôle to workers in many fields of social work. She gives 'useful lectures' in university extension courses for social workers, is an excellent leader of group discussions and helps with the training of social science students. She appreciates that there is an educational job to be done and is ready to interest herself in the wider field of social work. The main contribution, according to this writer, which a psychiatric social worker can make to the social services in the community is that of improving, by example and interpretation, the quality of social case-work, and the 'human relations job generally' which is being done by family case-workers, club leaders and the rest. The second, writing of a subject employed in a mental hospital, remarks that as a social worker she speaks the same language as social workers in other organizations and has the duty of interpreting to them the emotional factors in mental illness.

To judge by these reports, a good deal is expected by the community of a body of people upon whose time the work of the hospital or clinic in which they are employed must always have first claim. Considering the variety in age, experience and capacity existing among those who bear the name of psychiatric social workers we need not be surprised to meet with some severe criticism in the reports of certain referees. It is convenient to consider together the criticisms of a group of referees who have in common the absence of psychiatric training.

One line of criticism is that psychiatric social workers tend to become so much absorbed in their work that they have come to form too exclusive a body. This is a danger which they themselves recognize, and the remedy which they and their referees suggest is the same—to mix professionally and unprofessionally with those whose experience and outlook are as different as possible from their own. When, however, a referee suggests that psychiatric social workers think that they have entered 'a world apart', the context shows that the criticism is of another order. Similar complaints are voiced by several referees. One has heard them spoken of by other social workers as 'an arrogant lot', while another writes that the newly qualified 'often come out quite arrogant', to join professional colleagues a number of whom have adopted 'an Olympian attitude'. Another, not committing herself to an opinion on this point, refers to the reputation which psychiatric social workers have gained amongst other social workers for regarding themselves as 'super people with a clue to some inner mystery which others lack.' One referee has had experience of 'anxious, unstable and inexperienced' psychiatric social workers, who claimed as a right 'the confidence which in every group can only satisfactorily be won by individual merit.' Another has observed students of the Mental Health Course who seem to confuse their own importance with that of the profession for which they are training.

These are formidable indictments and the experience of those who make them gives their words much weight. Two of these indicate what their conception of psychiatric social work is. One with great experience in many fields of social service gives her views on what the difference would be between a job of social work undertaken by someone who had and someone who had not had a psychiatric training. Without the training, she suggests, the social worker would not be able to analyse a situation or relationship, or to detect abnormalities in individuals; she would be less aware of her own emotional reactions and of where she was going and how to get there. The psychiatric social worker, moreover, would be able to interpret to others 'how the world looks to a child'.

The other, an administrator, writes of her as able to take a more 'fundamental view of social tension' than is commonly found among general social workers. These can learn from her, provided that she can handle colleagues with the respect and tact with which she handles patients and that she shares their competence in and appreciation of social work. Referring to the influence for good or ill which a psychiatric social worker can exert in an organization for community care she describes her as a 'vital part not only of the clinical team but of the administrative and policy building mechanism, provided always that she has experience and judgment to win recognition in these spheres (at best she is the centre of a star formation).' She adds however that an anxious, inexperienced worker with a certain kind of 'infectious' instability or limitation, has, in her experience, 'by virtue of the same unique position, created more disharmony and waste of effort in every sphere than any other member of the team.' Not unnaturally, this referee is of the opinion that 'only the cream of ability, stability and good judgment should be accepted as students for the Mental Health Course.'

In an earlier chapter we described the psychiatric social worker going out into the community to discover how she could be used in the solving of some of the individual problems of war-time evacuation, and pointed out how easy it was for her to let herself be invested with magical powers. We wonder whether something of this kind of magic is not still at work. A course of training is established associated with psychiatry, a subject liable to exert a peculiar attraction and one towards which the eyes of social workers were already turned for a solution of some of their most baffling problems of case-work. Round this course is drawn a circle of a special kind of selection, in which the personality of the candidate is known to play an important part. It was perhaps almost inevitable that there should be some inflation in the ideas of those who passed through this guarded training and those who did not, and equally inevitable that the deflation, which was bound to follow, should lead to irritation in those who had set on a pedestal such patently human figures.

We have no means of estimating the extent of these misconceptions. Those both inside and outside the Mental Health Course, with other professional experience against which to measure it, will always have viewed the situation with a more sober eye. Those aware of the difficulties of recruitment and selection do not think in terms of 'cream', delighted as they may be when they meet it. Those responsible for training are forced to think realistically about what can be achieved in a course of a single session. With regard to employment the fact that in this still young profession demand has, for the greater part of its existence, considerably exceeded supply is recognized as involving dangers both to its healthy growth and to its reputation. There have been posts of a pioneer kind urgently needing to be filled which called for workers of long professional experience, but for which there has been no candidate available except a recently trained worker who, both for her own sake and the profession's, would have been better engaged in consolidating her training in a well established post in association with experienced colleagues.

It will be noted that the criticisms which we have quoted do not fall upon the psychiatric social worker as case-worker. We suggested in an earlier chapter that the emphasis placed on case-work in training, which we believed to be justified, could only be at the expense of other kinds of experience desirable in themselves. We should expect that the deficiencies of newly trained workers would show themselves rather in their understanding of the whole professional situation in which they have to find their place, than in the practice of specialized case-work, much as they will have to learn in this sphere also. This is borne out to some extent by the evidence of our study. Perhaps the most significant comment comes from a psychiatric social worker with considerable experience of co-operative work in community service, who remarks that psychiatric social workers seldom fail in understanding a patient, but tend to antagonize other workers through failure to appreciate the responsibility of the latter in cases where they, as well as the psychiatric social worker, are involved. This is important, since the latter's value as an interpreter between psychiatric and social depends on her understanding both the spheres between which she undertakes to mediate. Her understanding must embrace such hard facts as the probation officer's legal responsibilities in regard to his probationer, by which she herself is untrammelled. It is possible that her own concentration upon the psychiatric side of a problem leads to her giving too little weight to its legal and statutory and other practical aspects. 'It is all a matter of human relations' is not a satisfactory answer to every social question and can be exceedingly irritating.

If we are right in our belief that the psychiatric social worker regards herself as more comprehensive in the way in which she applies her psychiatric understanding than the psychiatrist, it is ironic that the criticism to which she is chiefly subjected, at least by 'lay' referees, is that of a failure in the understanding of colleagues beyond her own small profession. How is it that her psychiatric understanding, according to her critics, stops short at this point? Perhaps she is sometimes over-anxious to assume responsibility for the relationship with them or even for general relations in the professional group in which she finds herself. These are not responsibilities to be assumed except by people who are at ease with themselves, and have what we would describe as a confident humility about their rôle. In the absence of this quality arrogance, or the reputation for it, easily slips in and makes genuine co-operation difficult.

Some of us are guilty at times of using to those with whom we work an approach mistakenly regarded as ' psychiatric', through which 'by indirections' we find 'directions out', when a less recondite method would not only show greater respect for our colleagues but also be more genuinely 'psychiatric'. Such an approach may, not without reason, be resented as arrogant. An unnecessary display of professional terminology, which may sometimes represent a wish to underline the special value of our contribution when we are not quite clear ourselves where the value lies, may expose us to the same charge. Perhaps too psychiatric social workers as a body are apt to be too portentous about themselves in their genuine zeal for their profession. Some of us, as in other professions, are doubtless really arrogant; these in the nature of things will be likely to cause repercussions out of proportion to their numbers.

The referee who spoke of the reputation which psychiatric social workers had gained of regarding themselves as 'super people with a clue to some inner mystery which others lack', suggested that this feeling about them would tend to break down if training in general social work were to be improved. We believe that this is true and that the remedy will come in course of time; in the meantime an attempt to bridge whatever gap in understanding exists needs to be made from the side of the specialized training. This is not a matter of adding to an already overloaded curriculum, but of making use of every opportunity to awaken the imagination of students about the problems and responsibilities of people whose form of social service is different from their own. Such awakened imagination, not easy to rouse or tolerate, is not compatible with arrogance.

When a way has been found of sending out students from the Mental Health Course with the right kind of belief in themselves and a clearer conception of what they have to give as a result of their specialized training, newly qualified workers will be better armed against exorbitant expectations of others and less likely to be unduly concerned about their own professional status. Yet it would be unfortunate if, in trying to avoid an unpleasant reputation for arrogance, psychiatric social workers should refuse the responsibility which is in fact placed on their shoulders, not least by their severest critics. Their criticisms leave no doubt that they regard psychiatric social work as important and that it is for this reason that any shortcomings and indiscretions in those engaged in it give rise to real concern. It is reassuring to find that the referee who is the severest critic of those psychiatric social workers who do not reach the high standard which she sets for them writes of her subject, of whose work she has a deep but by no means blind appreciation: 'I think what stands out in my own mind is her humility, which enables her to learn constantly from others, but which in no way impairs her own confidence in what she can do. Her great respect for the capacity of individuals, her almost crucifying self-examination, which is not at all morbid. Her ambition for her work as apart from herself.'

ii

Criticism of psychiatric social workers does not as a rule distinguish between those whose contact with their social worker colleagues is made from the basis of posts in clinic or hospital and those in non-clinical posts in the open field of social service. It is to these, employed in 'community service' or 'community care', that we shall now turn. The terms are convenient but not easy to define. Our difficulty is increased by the fact that in community care under local authorities, which has largely replaced work under voluntary auspices in which the subjects of our study were engaged, a common way of using the psychiatric social worker's services has not yet, as far as we know, emerged. We can only indicate certain features which seem to characterize her part in community care in any conditions.

Like the work undertaken from hospitals and clinics it consists of individual case-work, administration, and work which, in a very wide sense, may be called educational. In community work the second and third assume a special importance and are likely to claim a larger proportion of a worker's time. The community worker must be able to appreciate a community's needs in relation to mental health and their relative importance, and to lead the community itself to work towards their fulfilment. She has a more direct and comprehensive responsibility than the clinical worker for promoting a better understanding of the general principles of mental health, and for combating the distorted conceptions of mental illness and the superstitious fears attached to it which still persist in the community. She works through direct education, among groups and through her case-work, which is always in the nature of a demonstration, and through a variety of individual contacts. She has special opportunities for encouraging those who need it to seek early treatment and to help others who have received treatment to readjust themselves to the community. To her there may fall the duty of supporting over long periods many whose illness is of a more chronic kind. In addition she provides an advisory service adjusted to the needs of those who would not, at least at the time in question, be prepared to consult a psychiatrist. The fact that the community worker is not usually under the same immediate psychiatric direction as her colleagues in hospital and clinic is a point which needs to be emphasized. It is one of the more compelling reasons why this work, while not in itself more skilled than that of workers in hospital or clinic, demands an unusual degree of experience and discrimination, and is therefore unsuitable for those who have just completed their specialized training.

Twenty-three subjects of our study engaged at some stage of their career in work of this nature. We tried to discover whether there was any type of personality to which the nature and conditions of community care were especially congenial. It might be that a difference of emphasis in the qualities demanded for clinical posts and community work would lead to a natural distribution of workers among them.

We found a small number whom our own impressions would have led us to assign either to a clinical or a community setting. But the records of these subjects' employment since qualification did not necessarily correspond with our impressions. They showed the majority of subjects qualified for as long as five years as having had a career in which work in clinic and hospital and some kind of non-clinical work appeared in different sequences. What we never found was an instance of community service constituting the whole of a subject's career since she left the Course.

We were interested in the different ways by which people entered and left community service and the different meaning the experience appeared to have for them. In some cases the period of community work was evidently incidental; in others it formed part of a more or less deliberate design. Two subjects left mental hospitals for community work early in the war, both influenced by a wish to undertake work more directly related to the immediate emergency. Both were glad to return when the opportunity offered to a hospital post and at this point one might have regarded them both as essentially clinical workers. Yet one, after a period of work in a mental hospital, left it once again for community care, this time to take up an administrative post in preventive work outside the field of mental health.

In other instances, however, we can have no doubt that the subject's real bent is towards clinical work. The period of community service then represents either a wish to enlarge experience or the disregarding of personal predilections in order to undertake work which urgently needs to be done. It is interesting to note how the workers whose preference is for clinical work adapt themselves to community service. One subject, who was led to enter community work by personal circumstances, dissociated herself from almost all its characteristic activities and confined herself to case-work. Another, whose senior position would not in any case have allowed her to withdraw in this way, showed the tendencies of a clinical worker in refusing to be drawn into expansive schemes of community education until she had raised the level of case-work among her social worker staff, and in enlisting local psychiatrists for consultation on their cases. This period of successful work in a type of post not naturally congenial was clearly valuable to the subject herself, yet it is not surprising to find her later in a post in a child guidance service, which she was combining with a post in research

Among the twenty-three subjects, two stand out as having carried highly responsible posts in this field for a considerable time, and as having, on the whole, found the work congenial. The first who before entering the Mental Health Course had been engaged in research quite remote from social or psychiatric subjects, passed from the Course to a research post held at a child guidance clinic, and stayed on as a clinic worker with responsibilities for the training of students. Service at a second clinic was broken by the outbreak of war and she entered the field of community care by way of war-time evacuation. The call to wider community service came three years later. In her new post of regional representative for the National Association for Mental Health there was scope for all the special abilities demanded of the community worker. When we saw her, some six years after she had entered this work, she made it clear that she regarded what she was now doing as the kind of responsibility which a senior member of a profession is under some obligation to assume. While she enjoyed the work's variety she found its lack of continuity distracting. Asked what she would consider an ideal job for herself within psychiatric social work, she described a post in a child guidance clinic which combined case-work with research, an ideal which in fact represented a return to earlier phases of her career. Here we would suggest is an example of sound professional growth, with roots capable of supporting the special responsibilities of community work. The second subject, who entered psychiatric social work at a considerably earlier age, represents a markedly different career, though one which seems to us equally satisfactory. After qualifying she spent one year in consolidating her training as the holder of a bursary in a county psychiatric service, passed on to the staff of the service and rose to the position of senior psychiatric social worker. This service formed a closely knit organization in a small area and by the end of six years she was feeling the need 'to break out into something wider'. The post in community care which followed had in it a pioneering element which appealed to her, and she enjoyed being thrown more upon her own resources than she had been in the psychiatric service. When interviewed she had left community care for research. She could not say whether this was the kind of work which would hold her permanently. It was something which she had to try out, in her eagerness to 'go deeper and deeper', for which her busy clinical and community posts had offered only the most tantalizing opportunities.

The Report of the Committee on Social Workers in the Mental Health Services (the Mackintosh Report), which appeared when this chapter was in process of writing, forces psychiatric social workers to consider the importance of consoliating clinical experience as a basis for any further responsibilities to be assumed as 'specialists' in the field of mental health. The Report envisages a future in which such educational demands will be made upon them that those concerned in selection might be tempted to attach a disproportionate value to what may be called gifts of communication. In selecting candidates for the Mental Health Course it has been assumed in the past that no qualities could compensate for the absence of those needed in case-work. It is true that an interviewer's report will sometimes note appreciatively that a candidate is likely to make a contribution to her profession on the educational side, but this has been regarded as secondary. The problem of the relation between the experience itself and its communication, which is of course an old one, is very relevant to the practical situation in which the profession of psychiatric social work stands at the present time, faced as it is with increasingly urgent need to make the most economical use of its members as 'specialists in their own field'.

The recognition of the value of the psychiatric social worker's services by the Mackintosh Report, because it is informed and not uncritical, is reassuring in a way which the demands for her services from employing bodies, some of them with a doubtful understanding of her functions, can never be. If arrogance, as so often happens, is based upon an uncertainty of worth, the Report should form a good antidote. Certain difficulties, however, suggest themselves. A general reading might lead to the inference that a certificate of a mental health course in itself guarantees the holder's capacity to undertake work of an educational and consultant kind.[1] Those who are themselves concerned in such training are very well aware that the awarding of the certificate represents a judgment based on the balancing of a student's achievement with promise, and takes account of a variety of gifts. Psychiatric social workers emerge from training at many stages of maturity, and development is possible throughout the whole of a professional career. The capacity to train, to advise, to stimulate and direct the work of others is something which needs to be reassessed at intervals. A final judgment should certainly not be made until time has been allowed for the digesting of one's own training and with some this may be a slow process.

It would be unfortunate if the wide educational duties laid upon the shoulders of psychiatric social workers in the mental health service should cause those workers to be under-estimated who have no special facility in expression, but all the qualities needed for good case-work. Such workers may always be ineffective in lecture or discussion. The most important part of training, however, takes place through a relationship between two individuals and the good case-worker necessarily possesses qualities which go a long way towards success in training of an individual kind. Some readiness and capacity to communicate the fruits of one's experience may reasonably be expected from any professional worker. Yet there are psychiatric social workers of the finest quality who not only have no wish to train others but to whom such work, as it is generally understood, seems to be definitely distasteful, almost,

[1] The Report recognizes, it is true, the need for those responsible for the supervision of 'trainees' to be specially selected (Mackintosh Report, par. 132).

for some at least, a violation. We believe that they are numerically rare, but, because they are also rare in the other sense, it is of the greatest importance that their influence should be felt among those undergoing training, whether inside or outside psychiatric social work. This should be possible without doing violence to their scruples and reserves. A student of some maturity and sensitiveness, given such a person as a supervisor, may learn more from simply working beside her than by more articulate and formal supervision from someone of poorer quality.

However the problem of training workers in this field comes to be solved, it would seem that there will have to be discrimination in the use of qualified psychiatric social workers, so that those newly qualified are not saddled with educational and consultant duties which might be detrimental to their own development during the first years of practice, as well as prejudicial to the confidence which the profession has won. The qualified psychiatric social worker who, as years go on, does not seem to be a suitable person to train others and yet has a wish to undertake it may present a difficult problem. For her sake and the sake of the newly qualified, and indeed for the stability of the profession as a whole, it is important that the position of the psychiatric social caseworker, as such, should remain in its own right an honourable one.

As the mental health services under the National Health Service Act becomes clearer in design and as the varied types of workers employed in it achieve a form of co-operation in which, it is to be hoped, they will find increasing satisfaction, what will be happening to the patient or potential patient, for whom all this organization exists? There are two related questions bearing closely upon the welfare and satisfaction of the patient for which the psychiatric social worker may be expected to carry considerable responsibility; first the sharing of cases among the various workers within the service and second the safeguarding of the patient's right to the greatest obtainable continuity of case-work.

In planning for the welfare of those in personal distress it is important to remember that each is an individual with a personality which may accord better with the personality of one rather than another among the workers who are available to serve his need, irrespective of their formal qualification or the extent of their experience. Keeping this always in mind it is nevertheless not unreasonable to ask whether there are not certain types of cases or certain kinds of work to be done, which can be regarded as suitable for workers with different degrees of psychiatric competence. This is a familiar question but might usefully be re-examinied in the light of new conditions. We can only draw attention to a few of the considerations which need to be borne in mind.

Two kinds of clients are likely to be regarded as the most suitable for referral to workers without specialized training, viz., those in whom the damage to mental health is slight and has been recognized at an early stage and those in whom, when they are brought to the notice of psychiatry, the results of the damage have been so deeply built into the structure of the personality that little interior change is to be expected. It is the second of these types of cases which we would consider here. The description covers the person who is often labelled a 'psychopath', to whom we referred in the last chapter. This condition, while accepted as lying within the sphere of psychiatry, seems often to present problems which are more obviously social than medical and therefore to be suitable for referral to social workers without specialized psychiatric training. In the present shortage of specialized workers it is tempting to think them so, since, if such patients are to be helped at all, they are likely to be time-consuming. Yet any experienced worker knows that few cases present more difficult psychiatric-social problems than these. It is just in this type of case that the recognition of the limitations imposed by the patient's state itself, which specialized training ought to give, may prevent not only wasted effort, but needless distress for everyone concerned. While this seems to suggest that such cases have a high claim to the service of the specialized worker, the history of work in mental deficiency should give us pause. The personal and social difficulties of an unstable mental defective, though differing in important respects from those of a person usually regarded as a psychopath, call for no less skilled handling on the part of a worker trying to help him, and demand to a special degree an understanding and acceptance of the limits beyond which development cannot be expected to go. Yet the patient, supportive work needed in the case of mental defectives has long been carried out by workers who, finely equipped as they have often been with the wisdom which comes from experience and with a special kind of compassionate concern for those they serve, have not, as a body, had the advantage of specialized training.

In thinking of the working of a mental health service it is not unpractical to see it as an act of co-operation in which human relations are in constant interplay. On them will depend questions of the most practical kind, above all the most economical use of available staff. Thus a case which might reasonably be regarded as beyond the scope of a worker without specialized training may in fact be undertaken by someone who is learning on her job, provided always that her personality is one which makes her acceptable to the client, that she has the natural aptitude for the work she has chosen and that she is able to make use of the experience and support of a specially trained worker, because the right kind of relationship has been established between them. Given all these, the patient may in fact receive from her not a second-best but the best possible service. Within this field of relationships the psychiatric social worker will not be able to avoid playing an important part. We have referred to her alleged shortcomings and also to the great expectations which she arouses. In the mental health service she will form part of an organization which will be in constant change and through which she herself must be prepared to be changed. Meanwhile it may be said without arrogance that her feeling of responsibility for certain values which her special training and experience have tended to foster, has never been more needed than in the present shifting scene. One of these is the significance of continuity in case-work.

It would sometimes appear as if psychiatric social workers were more aware than psychiatrists of what lack of continuity in treatment may mean to a patient. They deplore the fact that, in out-patient clinics especially but also in mental hospitals, patients seem to be passed from one psychiatrist to another without due realization of what the effect on the patient may be and so without due preparation for the change and even, in some cases, without due courtesy. There is a temptation to assume a rather superior attitude about this. Yet there has always been a good deal of discontinuity in the case-work of psychiatric social workers themselves, the inevitable result of the passing on of cases from student to student in training and of the considerable mobility of workers within the profession. It is unlikely that this discontinuity will decrease. If this is true it would seem that the time has come to try to gain a deeper understanding of what both continuity and discontinuity may mean for the client, so that both can be more understandingly allowed for and their effects brought under greater control.

Any exploration of the problems of continuity would need to include what continuity in case-work means for the worker herself. We believe that there would be general agreement about the importance to any case-worker of carrying a minimum of sustained case-work, even in conditions which make it necessary for her to delegate the greater part of her work or deal with it through more summary methods than she would choose to employ. To the psychiatric social worker sustained case-work is her earth, to which she must constantly return to draw professional strength to meet the increasingly varied claims which are being made upon her.

NOTE

ON PSYCHIATRIC SOCIAL WORKERS AND MENTAL DEFICIENCY

The Mackintosh Report refers (para. 71) to the 'negative attitude' towards work in mental deficiency found among students in social science courses, who nevertheless show an interest in psychiatric social work. It suggests as the remedy that the scope of mental welfare work should be enlarged. The Report also suggests (para. 124 (iii)) that provision should be made for more adequate theoretical and practical training in mental deficiency within the mental health courses. It may therefore be useful to consider the attitude towards work with defectives and the views about the teaching of this subject in the London course found in the group of students covered by our study. Since we did not include any question on mental deficiency in our scheme of interviewing, our material is not comprehensive. In what follows we shall indeed be drawing largely upon the statements of eight students, who had some experience of work with mental defectives either before or after taking the Course.

As far as it goes our study tends to confirm what the Mackintosh Report suggests, that work in mental deficiency, if it is to attract and retain workers, should form part of mental welfare work of enlarged scope. One subject, at a certain stage of her career as a psychiatric social worker, undertook a post in a voluntary association for mental welfare in a county where, at that time, no other psychiatric social worker was employed. At first her work was varied and included psychiatric out-patient clinics served by psychiatrists from a mental hospital. Later, however, a special psychiatric social worker was appointed to the mental hospital and a child guidance service was established in the county. It then became clear to her that the work of the voluntary association was likely to be confined in the future almost entirely to work with mental defectives. This certainly influenced her decision to seek another post. In this, where work at a mental hospital, in a child guidance clinic and with mental defectives was combined in about equal proportions, she stayed for over four years, leaving only to undertake a wider administrative post, and then with reluctance. Another, who had entered the course from work in a voluntary association for mental welfare with the intention of returning to work of the same kind, adhered to her decision. The work which she was invited to undertake on qualification had the additional purpose of demonstrating the value of psychiatric social work in two mental hospitals. Such work as she undertook with mental defectives was secondary, and was eventually given up when she became established as full-time psychiatric social worker in one of these hospitals. Another applied for admission to the Mental Health Course from a post in mental deficiency so wide that it included undertaking work for a mental hospital and a child guidance service. For this she felt herself quite inadequate without further training. In her case her original intention to return to her work in mental deficiency when she was qualified was deflected during training through her growing interest in mental illness, and from that time onwards her contact with mental deficiency has been confined to that common to workers in any mental hospital or child guidance clinic.

One young candidate entered the course after a year or more of experience with mental defectives. At the end of training, when it was felt that she still needed to work under some degree of supervision, she decided to return to mental deficiency work as assistant to a very experienced worker well known for her competence in the training of students. After three years of this work, with her confidence built up, she passed outside mental deficiency, and when interviewed was working in a mental hospital. The contribution of another subject to mental deficiency covered a much longer period. Entering the Course after two years in this work, she had no intention of ever returning to work with the mentally defective or sub-normal. Yet when, at the end of her training, she was asked to undertake a job of this nature she accepted it, her interest in this work, she suggested, being greater than she had realized. It was not till eight years later that she passed on to work with the mentally ill.

Of the eight subjects who before or after entering the Course had been engaged in work in mental deficiency three did not qualify. The admission of one of these, who was among the older candidates, was partly dependent upon the fact that she intended to return to her former post in this field. This she was able to do in spite of her failure to gain the certificate. The second who had also worked with defectives before admission, after leaving the Course held several posts in mental deficiency and was at the time of her interview employed as social worker to a large institution for defectives. The third, who had had no experience in such work before entering, was able to pass direct into training for work in occupation centres for defectives when, at a comparatively early stage, she withdrew from the Course on advice. When interviewed she had advanced since her second training to a post of greater responsibility and was obviously interested in her work.

Two of the eight subjects made comments on the teaching of mental deficiency in the London Mental Health Course as they had known it. They must be considered in relation to the remarks of others who appreciated the clearness of the teaching in this subject and valued the opportunity of visiting defectives in their homes with experienced mental deficiency workers. One of these two suggested that not only was there too little teaching on this subject in the Course but a tendency among the students to 'think it beneath them', an attitude which, she thought, was shared to some extent by the training staff. The other, looking back over a twelve years' career in which two of her posts had been partly concerned with mental deficiency, complained chiefly that the Course had not helped her to realize what a defective was like. When she entered her first post in a mental hospital she was not able to appreciate a diagnosis of underlying mental defect in the case of the mentally ill. When later she undertook the secretaryship of a local association for mental welfare, her knowledge of mental defectives had to be built up from the foundations.

iii

There remains to consider the passing of qualified psychiatric social workers to employment outside the field of mental health, a process which is termed 'wastage' when regarded from the standpoint of the field suffering depletion. In relation to psychiatric social work the term needs to be used with special care, as even our own small study shows.[1] Among the subjects there were some who had ceased to be technically employed as psychiatric social workers. These we shall consider later. Others, while still thus employed, did not seem to us to be firmly established there. To our questions whether they regarded psychiatric social work as the type of work for which they were best fitted and whether they felt well suited to their present job, a number of answers had a conditional character, which suggested restlessness or a lack of satisfaction in their work, though no regret for having undertaken the training. Some subjects saw themselves as trying out in the future other types of work within their own profession, but others seemed doubtful whether they would remain indefinitely inside its borders; a few had already explored the possibilities of work outside.

Our study showed two divergent trends. One might lead no farther than from clinic or hospital into community care in the field of mental health, though in some cases it led out into the broader field of general social welfare, where mental hygiene is to be found in its preventive rather than its therapeutic aspects. Work with deprived children in connexion with children's homes or as children's officer under the Children Act of 1948 represents this first trend. Such work is characterized by much administration, the leadership of one's social worker staff and wide social responsibility. This is a combination of functions which for some experienced workers has great attractions. The other trend is marked by a wish for an opportunity to undertake more intensive work with individuals, and for freedom from administrative duties. The responsibility involved, which is at least as great, tends to be narrower and deeper. This trend is in the direction of the psychiatrist practising as a psychotherapist. It is represented

[1] We are not giving special attention here to the group of qualified subjects withdrawn from salaried work as psychiatric social workers because of marriage and the responsibilities of a young family. Such information as we have about them and about those of them who withdrew at an earlier stage and have since returned, suggests that there are so many variables involved that only after making a special study (and this we are not able to undertake) could we draw inferences which would not be misleading. It is important to remember, however, that those who have been, or are still, withdrawn from salaried professional work may be carrying out, through discussion groups, lectures, writing or in other ways, educational work in mental hygiene which may have a special value and authority, because it draws both upon their professional assets and upon the personal experience which they are passing through at the time.

by the attraction of the work of a lay analyst and of a play therapist, both of which forms of work, unlike the type of employment referred to under the first trend, demand not only a personal analysis but a specific additional training. It does not necessarily follow that those who consider such a further training, or even undertake it, will eventually break with psychiatric social work. While in some cases this can be safely predicted, in others, where the main need is less a change of profession than an opportunity to go 'deeper and deeper' at whatever spot they are at the moment standing, psychiatric social work itself may be able to offer certain posts, especially in child guidance, which will provide the satisfaction they seek. We have examples of some whom, after a period of uncertainty, their own profession proved able to contain.

With these trends in mind we shall turn to a few of the subjects who, at the time of writing, are working outside the field of mental health in posts for which the qualification of the Mental Health Course is not required. For the first, her present occupation, that of a professional musician, has involved a complete break. There seems no need in this case to look for causes of dissatisfaction within the profession itself or indeed within the subject. During her six years' service in a child guidance clinic her work was of a quality that gained for her the highest rating from both her referees. Of how it felt to herself she writes: 'I think I was an adequate p.s.w., but music was always what I pined for. Failing music, I think psychiatric social work was what I was best suited for and, failing music again, I think I would choose to go back to it— probably the better for having satisfied what I yearned for.' In contrast to this subject, lost to her original profession through the growth of an overriding enthusiasm, we have another who made an almost equally drastic change of occupation but for very different reasons. After some years of service in clinical and community posts, she had come to be uncertain of her suitability for this work and evidently questioned the validity of her motives for entering it. 'I wanted to do something for others, to make up for all the "bad" things that I had done, although I did not realize until I was analysed that I had such guilt feelings.' We do not, as we hope we have made clear elsewhere, doubt the value of a positive wish to serve as a motive for undertaking social work; in this case however there are indications, most of all the subject's satisfaction in her present work, which point to a mistaken vocational choice.

This subject bore witness to the value of her training in all that side of her present work which is concerned with human relations. The same testimony was borne by others now engaged in professions other than social work, including the head-mistress of a large school in East London, a doctor in general practice and a medical student. In the case of the one subject who is practising as an analyst, the transition from many years of work with mothers in a child guidance clinic to lay analysis gives the impression of a natural and inevitable process, even though the Mental Health Course, in which she discovered her unusual gift for intensive case-work, was based upon a solid experience of general social work.

Among the subjects who have passed beyond the mental health field proper to the general field of social welfare, three are engaged in work directly concerned with children, with so large a proportion of administrative work that the amount of case-work which they themselves are able to undertake is very limited. Two, after working as psychiatric social workers for about ten years chiefly in mental hospitals, are employed as children's officers. The third holds a highly responsible administrative post in one of the large voluntary organizations for deprived children. Viewed from the point of view of 'wastage' her career is instructive. Entering the Mental Health Course with a considerable experience of work with children, she seemed a likely recruit for child guidance, though she herself had made no decision at this point. The special obligations of war-time led to her entering community care, which for a time postponed a decision. Her own opinion is that she is too 'unorthodox' to fit into a child guidance team. Her present post, therefore, outside the field of mental health but related to it on its positive side, and making full use of her accumulated experience and training, seems to represent a solution to a vocational problem for which the term wastage seems singularly inappropriate.

In tracing the rise of psychiatric social work in this country we described how, in the early days, many of those responsible for the teaching and supervision of the London Mental Health Course had received their specialized training in U.S.A. At present almost all psychiatric social workers on the staffs of the three training courses have received their training in Great Britain. This natural process is represented in our study by three subjects who are employed as tutors in mental health courses and by a number who are responsible to a greater or less degree for the supervision of students training in practical work. What our study does not illustrate is that psychiatric social workers appear to be increasingly used in educational work outside their own profession. In the list of members of the Association of Psychiatric Social Workers published in January 1951, supplemented by the list of April 1952, four are shown to be employed in connexion with the training of workers for the child care services established by the Children Act. Three are employed in social science departments of British universities, one as head of the department, while another holds a similar position in one of the Commonwealth countries. One holds a responsible post in the training of students, in an organization for general social work.[1]

In the present shortage of psychiatric social workers practising their profession and available for consultant and educational duties in the field of mental health, the transfer of any of these to other fields of work cannot be regarded lightly. This is especially true of such workers as are likely to be chosen for the educational posts which we have mentioned. Nevertheless, we cannot but watch with interest this form of 'wastage' and welcome it on several counts. We welcome it as a recognition that psychiatric social workers have something of general value to contribute beyond their own borders and are not considered too hidebound to make available the results of their specialized training and experience in a way that meets the needs of students preparing for work different from their own. It will be remembered that the critics whom we quoted earlier seemed to be calling upon psychiatric social workers to come out into the open, so as to enlarge their understanding of the problems of those engaged in other forms of service than their own and to practice the art of human relations in a larger professional world. Not a few are already gaining this invaluable experience and this should be constantly filtering back into the profession. If psychiatric social workers sometimes act as though they have 'entered a world apart', there is a steady movement in the other direction, sweeping them back into the wider world again.

It is important, even in an emergency, to preserve the distinction between 'wastage' which is due to something unsatisfactory within a profession, preventing it from holding its more gifted and experienced members, and 'wastage' which attests a profession's

[1] Cf. Appendix I, pp. 252–3, where however overseas members are excluded.

flexibility and growth. We recognize the existence of certain conditions which may lead to 'wastage' of the former kind; our study gave us some indications of them. Yet most of all it impressed upon us how complex the professional careers of individuals are and how wide a field is needed in some cases for careers to work themselves out, taking into account not only the greatest satisfaction of the individuals, but the greatest advantage to the community which they wish to serve.

CHAPTER X

PERSONAL DIFFICULTIES

i

THE subject of this chapter is one of the most important which we have undertaken to consider, as it is certainly one of the most difficult. It would be a simple matter if we could say that anyone who showed indications of personal difficulties during training or employment had slipped through the meshes of the selection net, that our present subject, in fact, was really one of unwise selection. It is by no means as simple as this. Personal difficulties are not the monopoly of 'failures' or 'near-failures' but are also found in students whose work during training and employment is of a very high standard.

We are using the term 'personal difficulties' in the sense of difficulties which arise mainly out of one's own personality. Obviously there are many other factors in professional success or failure. A student may withdraw from training because she finds it incompatible with the claims of her family or she may be unable to continue because of physical illness: In employment she may be faced with conditions which anyone would find unfavourable to good work. These difficulties do not come within our definition, but in all the cases we have mentioned personal difficulties may affect the way in which the individual handles the situation, even if they have had no share in bringing it about. We do not include inadequate intelligence in itself within the definition, yet the student who enters the course feeling seriously handicapped in this respect may suffer considerable emotional disturbance; or again, good intellectual ability may be masked during training by emotional problems. It is obvious that personal difficulties, as we use the term, have to be thought of relatively. We shall not expect anyone, student or staff, to be completely free from them. Into the training, as we shall illustrate later, come students who carry their difficulties in many different ways—disturbed students unaware of their existence; others who are well aware of them but are trying to conceal them without denying their existence to themselves; others again who show no obvious signs of personal difficulties but whose work is limited in a way which suggests their presence, deeply overlaid within a rigid personality.

Those responsible for training in psychiatric social work are sometimes regarded as people always on the alert for personal difficulties in their students, just as psychiatric social workers are sometimes thought of as expecting every child to be 'a problem child'. The criticism should not be lightly brushed aside. All who have taken part in such training must know how easy it is to anticipate personal difficulties and so to introduce an element of anxiety. In such an atmosphere it is hard for students to enjoy spontaneously what, after all, should be an interesting venture in learning, as many fortunately seem to have found it, in spite of the mistakes of their teachers.

An atmosphere of anxiety once engendered in the Course may spread beyond it. We think that it would be unfortunate if too much stress were laid at the time of selection upon the possibility that the training will stir up latent problems and prove an emotional strain. Nevertheless the possibility is a real one and in particular cases it may be wise to help a candidate to face this before committing herself. One subject spoke of the training as having been no more disturbing to her than if she had taken a course in dressmaking, 'perhaps even less so'. This is surely to 'protest too much'. The analogy is in any case misleading. The material on which the students of psychiatric social work have to learn is human material and consists chiefly of people who are themselves in severe personal difficulties. Supervisors of practical work always carry a double responsibility, for the welfare of the individual in need of professional help and for the provision of the best possible experience for students. It is a serious matter to take the risk that a student, who is herself known to be under the stress of personal difficulties, may work out her own stress through her relationship with those she is called upon to help professionally. A watchful attitude on the part of the supervisor is often fully justified. It is when it becomes a pervasive state of mind that it may distort the training from its original purpose.

Learning on human material is not of course peculiar to psychiatric social work and the problem of how far personal difficulties can be damaging to professional work enters into any profession which is concerned with human beings as individuals, notably into other branches of social case-work and into psychiatry. What makes psychiatric social work especially aware of its responsibilities in this respect, and possibly over self-conscious, is the fact that it has from the beginning insisted upon the importance of personality in the selection of candidates for training. It is not unnatural that those concerned in selection and training should give close attention to the question of what happens when candidates who have been admitted for training prove to be emotionally disturbed. In this way, through the twenty odd years during which training for psychiatric social work has been going on in this country, something should have been learned about the relation between personal difficulties and professional work which may have a bearing on the problem as it appears in kindred professions.

Our special study provided material on this subject no less valuable because we asked no direct questions to draw it out. We shall use this freely in the present chapter, although it will be easily understood that in presenting our illustrations we have been limited here to a special degree by the need to ensure that they shall not be identifiable. We are concerned, in any case, not with the essential nature of students' difficulties or how they originated in the depth of personality but rather with the way they showed themselves in the particular situation of training for psychiatric social work.

While personal difficulties are by no means confined to those who fail to qualify, it is among these that they tend to be brought into the open during training and so can be more easily studied. The nature of the difficulties and their manifestations vary widely. One feature, however, these students may be said to have in common—a sense of being in a false position in regard to the training itself. It seemed to us that subjects tended to deal with the uneasiness which this caused them in one of two ways, which itself threw light on their personalities and the kind of difficulties they brought with them. A small group tended to withdraw into a kind of dull bewilderment while a larger group tried to put a good face on things and to 'keep their end up'. These contrasting attitudes could be traced, to some degree, in the students' general bearing and behaviour, in their approach to the whole experience of learning and in their way of meeting the demands of practical work, particularly that of entering into a professional relationship with someone needing help. Both groups, the more passive and the more active, put up such defences against the discomfort of their position as to be, to a greater or less extent, incapable of using what the Course had to offer.

Turning to the reports of tutors and supervisors on the first group, we find that one student was 'in a complete whirl', another had periods of 'dazed depression' during which case-work was quite ineffective, while pathological conditions distressed her so much that she seemed to be 'enervated to the point of listless apathy at times'; another could not give her mind to lectures because she was 'too much taken up with her imagination'; another had periods when, 'present in the body but most unwillingly in mind and spirit, she had withdrawn to the greatest possible distance'. When these students applied for admission there was in every case some doubt among those who interviewed them about their suitability, and in some cases very serious doubt. One was described as 'enigmatic' and another as constantly sidetracking her interviewer when she tried to find out what she felt or thought about anything. In one case defensiveness appears as 'social adroitness'. In another candidate, who was severely disturbed during training although she had entered unaware of her own difficulties, the psychiatrist who interviewed her noted a degree of self-assurance which made him suspect 'over-compensation'.

In the second group, consisting of those who tried to put a good face upon their discomfort, we found that their attitude and behaviour often impressed others as inappropriate in students committed to a professional training. The bearing of some is described as artificial, affected or self-conscious, and this is sometimes reflected in a pretentious style of writing. One student, with a singularly contorted style, herself admitted that she was afraid to put things simply. In several we found an undue wish to please. One supervisor wrote of a student's 'extreme superficial pliability which is extraordinarily hard to deal with'. On the other hand, one is described as showing so little sense of propriety that those with whom she worked did not take her seriously.

Such students are unlikely to be able to give themselves disinterestedly to the interchange between client and worker. In the first group, when we found a student withdrawing from the impact of case-work, we had the impression that she was aware of what it might involve to enter into the personal difficulties of others, and could not face it. In the present group, if the same sensitiveness was present, it seems to have been more deeply overlaid. A supervisor reports on one student that she has a detachment which is 'not that of an easy professional relationship'. Of another it is reported that, when interviewing for a social history, she would take the withholding of information personally and try to extract it by frontal attack. Another, in her work at a child guidance clinic, is described as 'constantly preoccupied with her part in the case, or in the mother's reactions' (i.e., to herself).

The attitude of this group to learning is fundamentally the same in academic and practical work and shows itself as a tendency to manipulate things so that deficiencies are not brought to light. One supervisor wonders whether a student, aware that she is not doing well in her practical work, is playing for safety by evading issues which she is unfit to handle, so that, in spite of the supervisor's belief that she is essentially unsuitable, there is 'nothing concrete to report adversely'. Another student is described as fending off discussions with her supervisor by herself proffering 'frank and searching criticism of her work and personality', while seeming in fact to be very little concerned about it. On the academic side the tutor of the same student reports that her studies fail to develop, remarking that she 'aims to impress rather than to gain and marshal knowledge and deceives herself with verbal fluency'. Of a student whose aggression was only partly covered by an overcorrect manner, her tutor writes that she has good powers of criticism but that her expression of opinion is checked by deference. Her tutor, she thinks, should know best what she ought to do. These comments offer a striking contrast to the descriptions of free and eager learning characteristic of those students who found in the Course what they had been looking for and brought to it a 'heart at leisure from itself'.

The relation between the impression made by these students at selection and during training is much the same as with the first group. In all cases one or more of the interviewers noted traits which raised doubts about the candidates' fitness for psychiatric social work; some were admitted with a recognition of serious risk. The particular traits which caused difficulty during training were not always obvious at selection, though in retrospect it is sometimes possible to trace them in disguised forms in selection reports. Some of these illustrate well the individual differences among those who interview. Thus when an artificial manner was particularly marked during training, it has nearly always been noted by one or more of the interviewers at selection, but in one case a manner which struck others as artificial impressed one interviewer as 'gracious'. This is interesting because, in spite of her façade, this student's essential sincerity was felt during training even by some who found her manner irritating. It had also impressed her tutor in the Social Science Course, who knew her well. We cannot always assume that the interviewer who saw the candidate in the more favourable and positive light was necessarily taken in by a façade. It is equally possible that, with this particular interviewer, the candidate was able to lower her defences and show something nearer to her essential self.

An over-anxious desire to please, which showed itself in several cases during training, was only commented upon in one case at selection. This is worth noting, since one would expect the circumstances of a selection interview to bring out this trait to the full. In the case of two students, however, with whom this tendency presented a serious obstacle to learning during the Course, it is possible that it was present at selection but not recognized. Each impressed one of her interviewers with her objective attitude towards the kind of personal experience which one would expect her to have found distressing and humiliating to discuss. Looking back, with the knowledge gained during training, one is driven to doubt whether the 'objectivity' was genuine. We hope that it is not cynical to suggest that these candidates, in their 'objective' discussion of their own affairs, were conforming more or less unconsciously to their idea of what was required of a candidate for the Mental Health Course. A cruder form of the tendency to manipulate situations found in students of this group during training sometimes tends to appear in selection interviews as overt self-assertion. This is evidently a quality which makes a very different impression on different interviewers, who also, on their part, no doubt evoke from candidates very different responses. An extreme example is that of a candidate who assured an interviewer of her fitness to take the Course as soon as she entered the room.

The difficulty which students of this group were to experience during training in entering into a professional relationship with a client is usually represented in selection reports by comments on a candidate's lack of imagination about how people feel and think, her tendency to over-simplify personal problems and the unlikelihood that she will give confidence to people in serious trouble.

About one, described as emotionally timid and aloof as well as domineering, an interviewer suggested that she had always thought in terms of getting her own position clear intellectually and then putting it over to the other person, and of another that she tended to think of children as material for laboratory experiment. These seem such serious handicaps to the profession which the candidates were trying to enter that it would be hard to explain how they came to be admitted, were the interviewers always in accord on these points. We have seen that this is not always the case, and it is clear that the quality in question is not easy to assess. Where interviewers were in agreement in not finding it, one must assume that a risk was taken in the hope that the kind of sympathetic imagination needed might be developed through training.

The candidate's capacity for learning through the training is not often assessed directly in selection reports, yet an account of how a candidate conducted herself at an interview will sometimes point to just those attitudes which later prevented her from giving herself to learning single-mindedly. The description of a candidate as 'afraid to commit herself' and 'too concerned with the impression she was making to be able to discuss on a real basis at all' gives the essence of her difficulties as a student. While the risk of accepting this subject was fully realized, in another case it seems possible that certain danger signals were overlooked. This subject is described during training as 'rationalizing away' her mistakes and laying her failures outside herself. With retrospective wisdom, we can now note how the critical attitude towards agencies and individuals, shown at selection in her account of her past professional experiences, gave warning of just that resistance to learning and self-criticism which she was to show in the capacity of student.

Some of those who qualified had reason to believe that, during at least part of their training, their suitability for psychiatric social work was in question. Not unnaturally their behaviour sometimes resembled that of subjects who failed to qualify. The example we have chosen is of a subject whose attractive personality was felt by all her interviewers. It was certainly noted that she tended to be too hastily critical and there was some doubt whether she would profit by this Course. Nevertheless her adequate training and experience, together with her positive personal qualities, turned the scale decisively in her favour. Her career as a student was a chequered one. Sensitiveness to the feelings of clients was offset by some degree of aggressiveness when she met with hostility, and an eagerness to learn was counterbalanced by despondency and uncertainty about the value of the work she was training for. Her own account of her training is an easily recognizable subjective description of the experience as reported by others. She thought the Course too intellectual, at least for someone of her temperament; it had taken away her confidence and not only temporarily. She had felt that people had wanted 'to make something different' out of her, she never knew what. She was always trying 'not to be herself'. The academic work seemed to have no bearing on the practical; it made her feel like a 'split personality'. At the centre for work with adults, when she could not avoid consulting one of the medical staff about her cases, she 'made herself as small as possible and got away as soon as she could'. She summed up her general discomfort during training by saying that, in a Course where there was so much talk about relationship, no really trusting relationships were built up and there was no true friendliness. When she was interviewed for the study it was hard to believe that this was not someone who had failed to qualify.

Her training had undoubtedly proved an unsatisfying experience; in the sequel, external circumstances took a hand. Having gained the certificate she made up her mind to get a really good job and 'just show them', but apart from holding some temporary posts in psychiatric social work, she was prevented, first by the war and then by personal responsibilities, from putting her plan into practice. This is an instance where, following the line of her own thinking, one is forced to consider whether entering the Mental Health Course was not a false step for this gifted, intuitive person. What might have been done during training that was not done to reconcile her temperament with the demands which being a student and psychiatric social work itself made upon her is a crucial question which it is now too late to answer.

We should like to refer briefly to the training of two older students, well qualified academically, both of whom evidently found it hard to be students again. Unfortunately we have no subjective account of their experience since they did not take part in our study, but it is certain that both were affected by the knowledge that their suitability for psychiatric social work was in doubt from the time of their selection onwards. Each made a considerable impact upon those around them, staff and students alike. In case-work both tended to make their clients too dependent upon them and one is described as entering into her cases too actively and dominatingly. The most notable common feature, however, is the use they made of sessions with tutors and supervisors. The tutor of one found it difficult to get a free exchange of opinion, while her supervisors found discussion of cases hindered by a 'press of self-justification' or a need to describe her former work. This comment might have been written about the second, who presented the further difficulty (not unconnected with her special gifts) that she was apt to dramatize an interview in reporting it. The supervisor who saw in her the greatest possibilities suggested as a condition of her success as a psychiatric social worker that she should find herself a position where her tendency to display would be accepted —not an easy condition to ensure, one would think, in the profession she had chosen. It is interesting to note that this subject, after holding several posts in psychiatric social work, left to cultivate her talents in quite a different direction.

While the discomfiture of certain students is obvious to all those with whom they work, and may even be discussed by them with their fellows, there are others whose personal difficulties seem to be of a different nature and to represent a fixed personality structure. We may take an example from among those students who showed a markedly critical attitude during training. It need hardly be said that a critical attitude is not regarded as in itself indicating a 'personal difficulty'. There have been students who made excellent use of training, and who seemed unusually free from personal difficulties, who were frankly critical, and probably rightly so, of various aspects of the Course in their day. There have been some students, however, whose critical attitude was more general and destructive, in the sense that it tended to undermine their own ability to make the best use of training. In these instances it often seemed to represent a defence in the form of attack, in someone who feared the training as a challenge to a hard won inner adjustment, which had to be maintained at all costs.

The student in question was recognized on admission as competent and intellectually able. She had grown dissatisfied with her former work and one of her selection referees thought that it had not 'liberated' her powers. The Mental Health Course, she suggested, might be just what was needed. In fact, however, the impression of an indefinable something holding her back persisted. Comments from supervisors represent this student as intellectually rigid and as showing a tendency to impose her views upon clients by argument, as afraid to show her feelings and as apt, in case-work, to deny the existence of a problem. Her tutor saw her as someone who covered strong convictions under scepticism and so appeared cynical about herself and others. At the study interview such criticism of the Course as was made was sensible and practical, yet curiously stilted; it would not have suggested the intellectual ability which this subject is known to possess. It would be reasonable to suggest that the same 'indefinable something' which held her back in training has operated in her subsequent career. Nevertheless, her psychiatrist referee rated her work as A, although he admitted that the qualities which he valued would not be acceptable to everyone.

The theme of defensiveness which has run through the examples we have considered hitherto continues through the three which follow, but with striking differences. These subjects, when they submitted themselves for selection, were aware of the presence of severe personal problems and came to their interviews deliberately defending their secrets. One of them, when interviewed for the study, described how she had taken upon herself the responsibility of not revealing the difficult situation in which she was then placed, lest she should be subjected to a special scrutiny of her emotional state, a proceeding which she would now regard as reasonable. In acting in this way she was supported by a strong conviction of her suitability for the work, which surprised her on looking back. In spite of their defensiveness all three made a very good impression at selection. In one case, it is true, a psychiatrist interviewer raised the question of neurotic tendencies but only to put it aside.

During training two of the three showed their quality at once and found special satisfaction in work with mothers at the child guidance training centre. With the third it was somewhat different. When interviewed for the study, she hesitated to give an opinion on the training because she had been so personally disturbed throughout. At one of the training centres she had felt it necessary to protect herself from the approach of her supervisor to her personal problems; at some point during training she had sought psychiatric advice outside the Course. By the end she was 'beginning to see light'. In her case, anxiety made itself felt in her work, but even at her first training centre, when the strain was specially evident, her supervisor suggested that she might go further than some students whose work was at present more effective, and by the end of her second period of training she was described as making marked progress in all directions. The following miscellaneous comments, taken from the supervisors' and tutors' reports on these three students, suggest the qualities which may be regarded as characteristic of them all: 'feels no need to demonstrate her value', 'discussion of cases fresh and the results of sincere and independent thinking', 'seeks advice readily', 'good sense of proportion and of honesty', 'receptive in attitude', 'quick to recognize and profit by mistakes', 'fine detachment in self-criticism and in accepting criticism', 'very honest, understanding, imaginative person, lacking all conceit', 'seeks advice and suggestions and is very ready to act on them, but intellectually mature enough to use supervision in her own way'. The contrast with the face-saving attitude of some of the students who failed to qualify is complete. That students who were admittedly concealing severe personal difficulties could yet submit themselves so freely to the experience offered by the Course is significant.

The careers of these students after training need not be given in detail. All were rated A by their psychiatrist referees at the time of our study. The most important fact from our present standpoint is that all three, between the end of their training and the date of our study, had undergone a personal analysis, which they had entered upon independently of the Course, although two, when interviewed, spoke of the Course as something which had led them to it.

Our two last examples are introduced because they raise, in an especially clear form, the question with which we shall deal in the section which follows—the responsibility of the training staff towards students' personal difficulties.

The account we shall give of the first is taken chiefly from what she herself told us at her study interview, although it is occasionally supplemented from training reports. Her general approach to selection was rather wary. Her interviewers found her 'elusive', though one of them caught a glimpse of the unusual qualities which were to reveal themselves later. During the Course the 'chatter' of the students about the disturbing effects of the training meant nothing to her. Even when her case-work at the child guidance clinic stirred her own early memories, the discoveries she made were 'interesting and in a way amusing'. In the adult training centre, in direct work with patients, she was aware of a gulf between their personalities and experiences and her own, but there is no evidence that this distressed her seriously. She was supported throughout by discussions with other students and by her vivid intellectual interest in the academic content of the Course. By the training staff she was recognized as sensitive, 'possibly over-sensitive', and highly self-critical, but her achievement in all parts of the Course was high. A supervisor's comment, 'takes nothing easily but will probably tolerate strain', must be mentioned in view of what came after. It suggests an underestimate of this student's difficulties or at least an over-estimate of her ability to deal with them alone.

On qualification this subject obtained a post in a child guidance clinic, which she enjoyed. Her second post involved working with cases of severe mental illness. In this connexion it must be mentioned that her training had taken place in war-time, when it was not possible to give students more than a limited experience of such cases. In the new post she grasped for the first time that mental illness might develop from apparently normal backgrounds, and also the high incidence of 'breakdowns'. After the first inevitable anxieties of a new post had died down, she found herself subject to feelings of panic and somatic symptoms which developed into an illness of several months. Eventually the symptoms subsided and, after a holiday abroad, she returned to work. Her psychiatrist referee rated her an unqualified A at the time of the study. A short report which she wrote on her experiences deals with the question of whether anything could have been done within the Course itself to prevent the occurrence of this illness; we shall quote from this in the next section.

The second example need not be given in detail. This subject went smoothly through selection and was described as 'unusually easy to interview'. Her training was characterized by various forms of stress, in part related to war-time conditions, and some anxiety was noted by one of her supervisors. The general impression, however, was of an outstandingly balanced, self-contained and highly intelligent person. One supervisor writes that this student would prove valuable as a member of any clinic staff and that 'others would come to rely upon her really excellent qualities'. This prophecy was in fact fulfilled, but another side of things was revealed by one of her referees who saw her work as to some extent undermined by her critical attitude toward the profession she had chosen. In the referee's view she was neither 'a convinced social worker' nor fully convinced of the value of her special training, since her attitude to psychiatry in general was sceptical. 'Would it not have been possible', her referee asked in effect, 'for more scope to have been given for the display of these critical attitudes within the training period itself?' With this question we pass to our next theme, the staff's responsibility towards a student's personal difficulties.

ii

We have tried to make clear, while drawing attention to the important contribution made by many others to the training as a whole, that responsibility for its more personal aspect lies with tutors and supervisors. Consultation between them goes on throughout the year but is especially close when students change from one practical training centre to another and towards the end of the session. It occurs, of course, at any time when problems arise in connexion with a particular student. Personal difficulties tend as a rule to have their most obvious influence on practical work, but when they occur here it is not uncommon to find that academic work is also affected. The supervisor is dealing continuously with case-work, which is specially liable to activate such difficulties and to be affected by them. Her report, which forms part of the material on which the Board of Examiners makes its final decision, may thus have great significance for certain students. It is for her to communicate its contents to the student in the way most useful to her, and this calls for judgment and skill which, as we are well aware, has not always been shown. The part of the tutor in such a situation is important, both because it is often useful for the personal difficulties, brought to light through case-work, to be discussed also in the more impersonal setting of the academic training centre, and also because the tutor is in a position to observe, throughout the year, how the student adjusts herself to different centres in relation to the particular personalities of the supervisors.

The examples we have given in the previous section illustrate how personal difficulties are to be found among students at all levels of achievement. We pointed out, however, that among those who failed to qualify these difficulties were, through the very fact of failure, brought into the open and therefore more easily studied. The same applies to the responsibilities of the training staff and we shall therefore start by considering this group of students in the present context. We must turn back first to the phase of selection.

Tutors and supervisors, even when they have not themselves taken part in a student's selection, are apt to feel for it a corporate responsibility when doubts regarding her suitability begin to arise. The concern naturally felt over any mistake in professional selection is accentuated by the implications about personality which failure carries in such a training course as this. Influenced by such considerations, the staff will be likely to err on the side of delaying action too long, rather than of facing the student too hastily with her inadequacy. And indeed it is possible to make a good case for maintaining a watchful inaction as long as possible. Different students will obviously take a longer or a shorter period to settle down. Experience has taught that some students, after a very uncertain start, do make good if left to go at their own pace. One of these whom we interviewed for our study, who admitted to quite serious personal difficulties during training but was rated A in employment, told us that she would not have been able, during her time at the first training centre, to stand up to anything more searching than the quite general guidance which she in fact received.

There is another reason for waiting on events. The practical work in the two training centres, one concerned with the problems of children and one with those of adults, is different enough for it to be common for a student to make a somewhat different impression in the two centres; it is indeed rare for her to feel equally at ease in both. In the case of one whose work raises doubts of her suitability at the first centre, it is reasonable for her supervisor to be reserved in her judgment, waiting until the student has had the opportunity to try herself out in the second, under a different supervisor. If the work at the first centre has been below a pass standard, the Board of Examiners could withhold the certificate until she has completed satisfactorily a further period of training in this type of work. Occasionally a student passing from one centre to another may be told that she is virtually on probation at the second. This may prove just the stimulus needed in certain cases, but for someone whose confidence in herself is in any case precarious it may make the start at the second centre unfairly difficult. This is not a matter for routine procedure.

These are some of the arguments for giving play to a student's own capacity for adjustment with the minimum of outside interference and we think that they should be given full weight. Yet it would seem that in some cases this has been carried too far. Some students, knowing that a doubt about their suitability existed, would have been grateful if the staff had approached their problems more directly and at an earlier stage. Perhaps some of those who did not qualify would have agreed with one of the subjects of our study, who herself qualified with distinction, when she described 'a Kafkaesque air of mystery as though all-powerful, all-knowing deities were silently assessing the students'. For these students the weekly discussion of case-work had not been enough; what they had evidently needed was a more direct periodic assessment of their achievement and what it indicated about their fitness for the profession they had chosen. In such cases we must assume that the supervisors had misjudged the needs of the particular students. Perhaps their error was not unlike that imposition of freedom upon those who are not able to use it which we deprecated in relation to clients in an earlier chapter.

Whether rightly or wrongly timed and prepared for, there comes a point at which the students we are now considering have to learn the fact that they are not considered suitable for the training for which they have entered. How can this be done with the least damage and distress? Obviously the question needs an individual answer, but there are certain general considerations which apply in all cases. The Mental Health Course, which has clearly informed candidates from the first that their selection does not imply that they will ultimately qualify, cannot accept responsibility for the future of a student who does not gain the certificate. It has, however, a strong obligation, comparable to that towards the candidate rejected at selection, to limit as far as possible the damaging effects of failure and also to handle the situation in such a way that the positive values, which on their own testimony many non-qualified students have found even in an unsuccessful training, are carried over to the next phase of their careers. In some cases, it is true, it is hard to believe that the personal difficulties which contributed to the failure in this training will not form a serious handicap in any future work. In other cases it seems likely that, with greater maturity and in work of a different nature, the non-qualified student may not only prove adequate but also put her experience in the Mental Health Course to good use in some more suitable form of work. Perhaps the greatest danger, in view of the particular kind of attraction which psychiatric social work exerts in certain cases, is that other work may continue to seem a second-best; we saw some signs of this among the students whom we interviewed.[1]

It is then clearly desirable that the non-qualified student should leave the Course with the feeling that the judgment made there about her and her achievement relates to one particular kind of work. Perhaps a frank avowal to all students on admission that knowledge has not yet advanced far enough for a positive assessment of a candidate's suitability for psychiatric social work to be made with any certainty, and that only experience within the training course can decide this, would help to ease the situation in advance. Moreover, a genuine belief in the positive value of other types of work is essential for any tutor or supervisor who hopes to be of use to the failed student in the difficult adjustment which faces her.

We have given instances of students of great ability and integrity who, as far as the Course was concerned, deliberately carried their own burdens of personal difficulties and whose development seems to have justified them in their decision. It appears to follow that in their case at least the training staff was also justified in not pursuing such evidence of tension as they observed. We would ourselves strongly uphold a student's right to self-direction, within the general purposes of the training and within the safeguards necessary to ensure that the clients through whom she gains her professional skill receive good service. These are obviously not easy conditions to ensure.

Apart from this, however, our study reminds us that, unless tutors and supervisors keep themselves constantly aware of individual needs, they may miss what might be called tacit appeals, especially on the part of the apparently self-contained and often able student. What these students have wanted from tutor and supervisor has not always been a direct approach by them to their personal problems. The subject already referred to who became

[1] Of the twelve non-qualified subjects about whose after-careers we have information the first jobs of several were admittedly taken as stop-gaps. Among the group as a whole there had been considerable changing of jobs before it settled into the pattern in which we found it. At that time two married subjects, one with a young child, were not in salaried employment. Three were working with mental defectives, one was in social work abroad; three were employed in direct work with children and one was about to start training for this work; one was temporarily acting as secretary to a doctor and the last was acting as managing director to a small firm, a type of work of which she had had experience.

seriously disturbed when faced with severe mental illness in her second post writes as follows:

> 'The two factors which stood out which I think might have been helped during the Course were (*a*) feeling completely isolated and convinced that this was a unique experience and must prove that I was entirely unsuitable to be a psychiatric social worker (also resentment that none had discovered my lack of balance before and stopped me knowing what I now know and therefore could not undo), and (*b*) feeling that my will had lost control and that I had no defences and little reason to combat my anxieties.'

She added, however:

> 'It is extremely difficult to know how the Course could have helped. Stressing the universality of the minds that get out of proportion and produce mental illness is, I suppose, one way, but this one never takes in unless one has experienced it. . . . I probably read it and was told it often enough, but it was almost impossible to apply when I was buried in my own state.'

It will be noticed that the remedy suggested is an intellectual one. To the supervisor the question is rather whether, within the relationship of student and staff and through case-work itself, even with the limited material available, the student might not have been helped to realize mental illness as something more than an intellectual concept, and to have made use of the supervisor in the process of facing this.

A subject who suggested that members of the training staff tended to throw up defences against students' personal difficulties on second thoughts changed her ground. The defences, she believed, were really her own, thrown up because she feared that the admission of personal difficulties might be taken as proof that she was unsuitable for psychiatric social work. This in itself suggests not only a misunderstanding but some failure in availability on the part of the staff.

When a subject comments on the tendency of supervisors to discuss case-work only in terms of relationship and mental mechanisms and to sheer off when students wish to discuss it in terms of philosophy and religion,[1] she is making an important general

[1] An article by Margaret Tilley, 'The Religious Factor in Case-work', has a bearing on this matter. *British Journal of Psychiatric Social Work*, 4, October 1950, pp. 54–60.

criticism, which may also cover a more personal one. The explanation for such an attitude is likely to vary from supervisor to supervisor. In some cases, for example, the attitude may be based upon a definite view about what training in case-work should and should not include; in others some more personal difficulty on the supervisor's side in discussing these subjects may be the chief determinant.

Tutors and supervisors naturally differ in their readiness to approach without invitation the personal difficulties of their students, so that the material, contributed by our subjects, represents a difference of experience. A certain number of subjects questioned a supervisor's right to 'probe' into students' personal history, though one implied that she considered it sometimes justifiable if it arose directly out of case-work. Some spoke of this kind of supervision as something against which one would obviously defend oneself. Two older students commented on its disturbing effect on younger members of their group although they themselves were not affected by it. We cannot from our study judge the extent to which these differing views are held. We asked no direct questions bearing on the matter and we recognize that it is one which some subjects would hesitate to discuss with us freely.

We have emphasized the importance of safeguarding the educational nature of training for psychiatric social work. The distinction between education and therapy is a real one; in the past the idea that the line between the two might become blurred would not have arisen. Yet anyone engaged in this training will know that in practice it is impossible to exclude from her dealings with certain students something which, if we are honest, we must recognize as akin to therapy. It is for this reason that we believe that the distinction should be preserved.

We have indicated how in the preparation for psychiatric social work in this country it is recognized that a year's specialized training will not result in a finished product of a certain type. Allowance has to be made among other things for individual tempo of growth and for the influence of continuous personal experience outside the course. It is in keeping with this conception that no specific provision is made for dealing with students' personal difficulties within the training. In Virginia Robinson's *Dynamics of Supervision under Functional Controls*[1] we find described

[1] Robinson, Virginia P.: *The Dynamics of Supervision under Functional Controls*, University of Pennsylvania Press, 1949, pp. 83, 84, 123.

an American method which brings out the British way of training in startling contrast. In the two-years' Course, regarded as a 'time-form within which movement takes place', the 'pressure to finish, to accomplish within the time limit, at the same time the fear of ending and of not being ready to end, operate in every task and in every time-limited relationship.' The supervisor's task is to 'break up a peaceful interval by holding the student to a fresh realization of problem in order to engage him in a new and deeper learning struggle.' To the argument that students who are slow to move forward in the Course so carefully marked out for them might make up later in working experience, the writer replies severely that 'to leave it to that, for the supervisor who is in this experience with him would be evasion of what is between them.' In comparison with such an athletic conception of training, to suggest that the fundamental responsibility of the training staff in their individual relations with students is that they should be available to them can hardly appear as anything but an 'evasion'. It does not seem so to us; moreover the kind of availability we have in mind demands on the part of the staff a degree of perceptiveness and wisdom certainly not less than would be called for in a more precisely regulated form of training.

It will sometimes happen that a student will discuss with her tutor or supervisor difficulties of a kind that suggest that she is in need of psychiatric advice, and that the best service which can then be rendered is to help her to accept this. Here at least is an opportunity for anticipating the fear, or allaying it if it should already exist, that the presence of psychological difficulties, even severe ones, necessarily makes a person unsuitable for psychiatric social work. When a student is in need of the help of a psychiatrist, the question arises whether such help is to be sought outside the training or whether provision is to be made for it within the Course itself. We are assuming here that the student remains in training, though it might well prove desirable for her to stand down temporarily if a period of psychiatric treatment should prove necessary.

The question has to be considered against the background of British education as a whole. It is certainly not an accepted custom, even though instances of it may exist, for psychiatric treatment to be provided within the educational system itself, whereas in U.S.A. the provision of a psychiatric service for students within a university, if not widespread, is at least an accepted idea. If the training courses in this country were to provide such a service, it would be on the grounds of the special nature of the work on which students are engaged during their training. However it may be in the future, at the present time in this country people do not as a rule consult a psychiatrist without being aware of fairly serious psychological difficulties.[1] To associate psychiatric help with training for psychiatric social work seems to imply in advance that such difficulties are anticipated to a serious degree among those who enter it, and to confirm the idea already too widely held that the psychiatric social work is something strange and set apart. It is for these more general reasons, as well as in consideration of the best interests of individual students in need of personal treatment, that we hold the opinion that such treatment should not be undertaken by those already concerned with training.

Psychiatric help within the Course has been drawn on indeed from time to time and we know very well from experience that a psychiatrist associated with her training can be of great use to a student, through what might be called psychiatric counselling as distinct from treatment. In addition, supervisors will themselves consult such psychiatrists when concerned about the influence of students' personal difficulties upon their work. Several of the referees of our study advocated that the training of psychiatric social workers should be more in the hands of psychiatrists than it is at present. If this comes about it will be interesting to see its bearings upon the question of psychiatric help for students in personal difficulties. We cannot usefully speculate without knowing the form of the training which the referees have in mind. We would suggest, however, that even in a scheme in which psychiatrists took more responsibility for students' case-work, and so became more aware of the personal difficulties which their work revealed, it would be no less desirable than it is at present to maintain the distinction between education and therapy in all relations between students and those responsible for their training.

iii

One of the psychiatrist referees of our study suggested that there was a tendency in the Mental Health Course to select away from

[1] The question of whether a personal analysis should form part of the training for psychiatric social work is of course a different matter. We have touched on the question in Chapter V.

the sensitive, intuitive candidate. He spoke in the highest terms of the subject whom he was assessing, as someone whom he valued as a professional colleague, but she was 'highly strung' and had had various physical ailments which might have been psychosomatic in nature. He was not prepared, however, to describe this as limiting her work. 'What she gains in sensitivity may mean more for the work than what is lost in instability.' Another psychiatrist referee placed the emphasis rather differently. For success in psychiatric social work there must be, in his view, a degree of instability or neurosis, but also enough fundamental stability to stand up to it. 'The best types may be those who have been in a fearful muddle and have had an analysis.' The subject whom he was assessing had come through her 'muddle' and could now 'stand anxiety without cracking'. Her work was of a high standard, especially her case-work, yet looking back the referee was doubtful whether he would have admitted her for training if he had been responsible for her selection, and pointed out how important it was to recognize the qualities which often lie within the apparent 'rigidity' of an introverted person.

Here we have two psychiatrists, both with experience of selection for the Mental Health Course, who see in a candidate's disabilities not necessarily a reason for rejection, but rather a potential asset for the work she wishes to undertake. But discussions on selection will often reveal the presence of a different school of thought. Signs of neurotic tendencies or emotional instability, even a history of psycho-therapeutic treatment reported as successfully completed, will arouse in its adherents suspicions about the candidate's motives for wishing to take up the work and strong doubts about her suitability. The difference between the two schools lies partly in the readiness to take a risk. The 'highly strung' person, or one who in the past has been in need of psychiatric help, might be assumed to be somewhat more liable to be unduly affected by the strain of work such as this, although we do not know of any conclusive evidence that this is true. The issue between the two would be whether or not the risk was worth taking. The two referees whom we have quoted obviously so regarded it, believing that, through taking the risk, recruits might be gained for psychiatric social work with qualities or a type of personality which they particularly valued. It is obviously possible, however, to hold a different view about the kind of person needed for the work. A profession in which one is largely concerned with unstable people and their problems might seem, on the face of it, to call for a special degree of stability in those who practice it and so need to be recruited only from among those whose mental health is above suspicion. This is indeed the common-sense view, yet a supervisor trying to awaken the imagination of a student so 'normal' that between her and even the most mildly neurotic patient there seems to be a 'great gulf fixed' may sometimes be driven to question it.

What the material of our study suggests, and wider experience confirms, is that the presence of personal difficulties, even those of quite a severe kind, is of much less importance than the attitude towards them of the person in whom they occur, which depends in turn upon the general structure of the personality. A person with such difficulties may become a danger in psychiatric social work or, alternatively, be capable of work of a quality beyond the reach of someone who has never experienced them, according to what she feels and does about her own problems. In studying those students with personal difficulties who were regarded as so unsuitable for psychiatric social work that they failed to qualify, we saw certain tendencies which seem to have formed an essential part of their personalities, whether their response to training was more active or more passive. In the one group we saw a tendency to cover deficiencies and to put a good face on things, which diverted them from coming to grips with their difficulties and in some cases prevented the training staff from establishing with them any real relationship. The evasion of the other group took the form of confusion and withdrawal, but made them no less inaccessible to educational help. Case-work, involving a sincere relation with another person, was understandably threatening to all of them.

When, on the other hand, we consider certain subjects who showed themselves undoubtedly fitted for psychiatric social work yet carried during and after training personal difficulties which were in some cases serious, we are impressed with their fundamental honesty, with an inner freedom which allowed them to face their own problems and yet keep intact an imaginative sympathy and an ability to establish sincere relationships. Some of them by no means wore their hearts upon their sleeves during training, but they were not concerned, like many of the failed students, about covering deficiencies. The impression they were making on those around them did not seem to interest them. They were thus able, in spite of the claims which their personal difficulties must have made upon them, to make use of the whole experience of the Course and, what is perhaps especially remarkable, were apparently able to place themselves freely at the disposal of those they were trying to help. They usually made good use of tutors and supervisors but were not dependent upon them. Several of them described how, even when they and their supervisors were not altogether compatible, the learning process through case-work still went on.

Out in the field of employment certain of these former students, some with and some without the help of a personal analysis, showed a steady all-round professional development. Others were noticed by those with whom they worked to show limitations which were inconsistent with their general capacity, notably a certain holding back in case-work, which made it seem more superficial than it should have been. We think of two who took part in our study about whom this would, to some extent, be true, but about whose value as psychiatric social workers there could be no possible doubt. One has, and one has not, undergone a personal analysis. In these subjects, as in some others, where personal difficulties seem to have been faced but not resolved, one is aware of an understanding of mental suffering which has a special quality, an understanding which is catholic in its conception of what constitutes mental health and leads to its appreciation as something hard to win and hard to maintain. These may have their own part to play among their professional colleagues.

In bringing together in one chapter such a variety of personal difficulties and in making such extensive use of the records of those who failed to qualify, we may have created an impression that the Mental Health Course is something which involves constant strain and stress. We hope that other chapters counteract this. In any form of education, but especially one concerned with understanding and helping human beings, staff and students alike must make use of their personal experiences. These may have been stimulating or humdrum, pleasurable or saddening, reassuring or distressing. For the most part adults are able to assimilate new learning to the experiences they bring to it and their education, in the widest sense, is thereby enriched. It may also happen, however, that the demands which the Course makes upon thought and feeling may fall heavily upon some individual at a particular time, forming a burden hard to carry. This may be the result of passing circumstances in a student's life outside the training or of the activation of personal difficulties of long standing by the training itself. Nevertheless we believe that, by the great majority of those who take part in it, the training tends to be remembered as offering the same steep cliffs, sloughs of despond, level stretches and quiet valleys of contentment as belong to any educational pilgrimage. We have taken this for granted in writing this chapter and we think that it forms the greater part of the story.

CHAPTER XI

ENDS AND MEANS

THE nature of our subject led us to think about the way psychiatric social workers regard their work. The words of one of the psychiatrist referees will serve to open the discussion. On the subject of selection he writes: 'I would be inclined to view with suspicion a candidate who appeared desirous of taking up social work service with a sense of mission. Other things being equal, I would prefer the careerist to the missionary. . . . Provided a candidate showed evidence of being conscientious and desirous of giving a little more rather than a little less service, I would be inclined to favour the attitude of what I would call benign scepticism than blind faith in the value and importance of the work.'

It would of course be misleading to treat the term 'mission' as synonymous with 'vocation' or 'careerist' with 'professional'. Nevertheless the writer of this passage starts us thinking about the theme of vocation and professionalism, which runs elusively through our material and has indeed formed one of the main sources of controversy since the early days of professional training. We wonder whether it would have occurred to the writer of this passage, a medical superintendent of a mental hospital, to write in the same way of other members of his staff—of psychiatrists, for instance, or of psychologists, if his staff included them. We have met among psychiatric social workers something like a puzzled envy of the psychologists with whom they work, who do not feel responsibility for the running of a clinic and seem to keep themselves free so easily to follow their specific functions, undisturbed by any conflicting ideas about what these functions are. Perhaps one always tends to see another person's problem as less complicated than one's own. Yet there is good reason why the attitude of the psychiatric social worker to her own work can never be a simple one.

The roots of social work are to be found in a conception of personal service which has in the past, more often than not, been the outcome of religious faith. In the general body of trained social workers to-day the religious motive is not consciously present; the history of the probation service illustrates a movement away from a missionary origin. With the individual social worker it is a different matter. Her choice of such work may be based upon religious motives, and upon a sense of being 'called' to take up such work which is vocational in the original meaning of the word. There is nothing, we believe, incompatible between such a sense and professional loyalties. Apart, however, from the position of individuals, social work as a whole has retained something of a special kind, felt by the social worker and ascribed to her by others, which some would prefer to call simply humanitarian but others feel to be religious. This can be disturbing just because it is not clearly identified.

Margaret Mead in *Male and Female*, approaching the question from the special standpoint of her book, writes: 'Between the two wars there was a marked decrease in the willingness of women to enter those fields which had been ear-marked as fields of "service"; that is fields in which the bad pay and heavy work were supposed to be ignored because they gave opportunity to exercise womanly qualities of caring for the young, the sick, the unfortunate and the helpless. This whole trend towards the professionalization of service fields means a shift from an occupation to which one gives oneself —as a woman still does in marriage and motherhood—to an occupation to which one gives definite hours and specified and limited duties.'[1] She draws attention to the paradoxical situation which has arisen. 'Even social workers, every hour of whose working day must, if they are to do their chosen tasks, be devoted to warm helpfulness, will defend their choice of a career because it is interesting or one in which women can do well. Only with many apologies do they now admit to a simple desire to help human beings.'[2]

It is interesting to compare this with the results of our study. This apologetic tone was certainly present at times and two subjects illustrate especially well the difficulty which people have, in this analytical and debunking age, in expressing simply any motive for

[2] It is worth noting that in the profession of medicine it is just this kind of unlimited self-giving which is imposed upon its practitioners by the Hippocratic oath.

[1] *Op cit.*, p. 305.

their choice of work which might suggest altruism. It is obvious how difficult it was for the first of these to make her confession. She writes: 'It sounds awfully "pi", but if this is more or less in confidence, I wanted to do as much as I could to lessen the misery of the world and psychiatric social work seemed to me the most helpful way of doing it.' Another writes of psychiatric social work: 'It met me in the two ways I am "called out". It seems silly to describe these ways thus, but I can do no better—I wonder about people and I love people.' When, however, subjects were asked to mark on a list of motives for applying for training those statements which were true of themselves, this difficulty did not seem to have been felt unduly. Statements were included which, combined, embodied the idea of expressing oneself in personal service. One which read, 'I wanted to help individuals undergoing mental suffering', was marked by thirty-five out of the seventy-nine subjects who completed the schedule. The other which read, 'I believed I had some natural ability for understanding and helping people', was marked by forty-seven, the highest score of any single statement except that of 'I wanted to qualify myself for psychiatric social sork', which was marked by forty-eight. Presumably the fact that we did include the statements in the list, and so at least recognized the possibility of such motives, was reassuring.

We quoted Margaret Mead as referring to 'a shift from an occupation to which one gives oneself—as a woman still does in marriage or motherhood—to an occupation to which one gives definite hours and specified and limited duties'. The transition from total commitment, the characteristic of religious vocation, to the division of one's life into working life and personal life, raises for the social worker the problem of the relation between the two. For the psychiatric social worker the problem is particularly urgent, depending in her work, as she does to so marked a degree, upon the disciplined use of her own personality. One of our subjects gave an account of her career which illustrates the conflict between the demands of professional and personal life. She described how she began as a social worker with strong professional ambition. This waned with the development of a rich personal life until at the time of her interview, when to advance professionally would demand from her the expenditure of more time and energy, she had discovered that she was no longer prepared to be 'a hundred-per-cent social worker'. We may compare the career of another subject who, in remaining for many years in a post which many would regard as offering little scope, is influenced by a personal life which makes her singularly free from emotional dependence upon the work she is doing.

Emotional dependence upon one's job is rightly suspect when this involves direct relationship with individuals. When candidates are interviewed for selection it is reasonable to try to discover whether the work they propose to take up is in the nature of a compensation for a meagre personal life. Psychiatric social work has a natural attraction for people who are to some degree aware of a poverty in their own lives and seek to remedy it obliquely through their profession. This is a matter about which it is very difficult to form a judgment at the stage of selection. We have known students admitted for training whose natural shyness and reserve have limited their personal contacts. Given, however, a natural warmth towards people and a sensitiveness to their needs, such a student may find herself in case-work in a surprising way. The confidence this gives her may lead to a general blossoming of personality, which can hardly fail to lead to freer personal relations. It would be a pity to make a bogey of the satisfaction one feels in using personality in one's job; such satisfaction is surely the basis of all good work in a profession such as this and is a very different matter from the exploitation of one's clients for one's own emotional needs. This is a question about which those training for psychiatric social work can easily become confused and distressed.

One might expect that the greatest safeguard against undue emotional dependence upon one's work would be marriage and motherhood. The material of our study gives us little help on this point. In an article embodying the findings of the Parents' Group of the Association of Psychiatric Social Workers entitled 'Home Versus Career', the question of the enrichment of professional work through the experience of marriage and motherhood is unfortunately not discussed. References to their professional work by some members of the Group seem to over-simplify the problem and sometimes to treat professional responsibilities somewhat cavalierly. One contributor is quoted as remarking: 'The result of Social Science andMental Health training is that most psychiatric social workers make a virtue of overwork. Since I have cured myself of this attitude, I find no difficulty (except in infrequent emergencies) in keeping to official hours. . . .'[1] It should be noted that overwork and failing to keep official hours are not the same thing.

[1] *British Journal of Psychiatric Social Work*, 3, 1949, p. 37.

Conditions in social work in general tend to make the reasonable limitation of hours more difficult than in work of some other types, quite apart from the question whether the people who enter it are themselves prone to this kind of excess. We do not know whether among social workers in general overwork is especially characteristic of those who have received psychiatric training; a few of our referees, it is true, mention it as a failing to which their subjects are prone.

The humanitarian version of a sense of vocation in regard to one's own work may perhaps be rendered as a sense of obligation to make the best use of one's capacities for the welfare of one's fellows. The first of these elements sometimes appears in the form of self-expression. We should like to illustrate the interaction of the two from the record of one of the subjects of our study. At her study interview she described how, when she applied for admission to the Mental Health Course, she was seeking work that would really give her satisfaction ; she was so preoccupied with this quest that she presented herself for selection without defences. On the other hand, the psychiatrist who interviewed her made no comment on this, but noted that her decision to take up social work was influenced by the motive of 'doing good', giving no opinion on the motive itself. As a student she soon proved her essential fitness for the work, and, once launched on her career, showed a fine balance between her need to develop her special capacities and her sense of obligation to meet the existing need for her services. Each step in her career seems to have been taken with both elements in mind. With a strong preference for intensive work with individuals, in which she has taken her own measures to increase her competence, she accepted, as an experienced worker, the obligation to shoulder administrative work, although she has no taste for it and carried it out at a considerable cost to herself. The balance which she has achieved between the two main motives, self-expression and service, is suggested by the comment of her psychiatrist referee, who described her, when she was filling an administrative post of great responsibility, as 'giving security to everyone', including himself.

The balance is not always so well preserved. Sometimes we seem to catch a glimpse of what might be called a 'mystique' of case-work, undertaken as a satisfying pursuit in itself and only rather tenuously related to the needs of the community. Yet, in some instances, the excellence of the case-work would seem to justify this kind of exclusive concentration and to constitute the individual's best form of service. When therefore a psychiatrist referee writes of the psychiatric social worker's use of her 'most highly elaborated technique' as 'an entirely personal gratification', this is surely to over-simplify a very complex matter.

The responsibility of the individual professional worker in relation to that of the profession to which she belongs raises many wide issues. There is the question of jobs needing to be done. There is also the fact that for most workers it is desirable to obtain varied experience before settling down to the type of work for which they believe themselves best fitted and which is most congenial to them. Yet there are some who, from the beginning, with impressive single-mindedness, are convinced that they can make the best use of their particular gifts in one particular kind of service. For these it would seem legitimate to seek within their profession for the highly specialized work which attracts them; to balance them there are always likely to be workers who prefer wider fields or changes in type of work. Highly specialized posts, however, are never likely to be common and most workers will have to undertake some duties for which they do not feel especially fitted and in which they are not especially interested. It would be unfortunate if these were undertaken with reluctance or in a spirit of depreciation, as it would be unfortunate if workers in one type of psychiatric social work should regard any other type as inferior. The safeguard seems to be for the profession as a whole to accept responsibility for meeting a certain kind of social need, but only if individuals feel their membership as a reality. Yet, in this country at least, the nature of this need, as well as of the specialized service which psychiatric social work has to offer, is far from clearly understood and while this is so, many questions depending on it must wait for an answer.

ii

Throughout this book we have applied the term profession to psychiatric social work as a matter of convenience, not knowing any general term which describes it more justly. Since, however, we have expressed a hope that our present study may have a bearing upon some of the problems which characterize other professions in direct contact with human beings, we are bound to pursue the matter further. In doing this we would not be thought to imply an isolation of this work from social work as a whole, or any branch of it.

A study of the professions, by Sir Alexander Carr-Saunders and P. A. Wilson, published in 1933,[1] while it makes no reference to social work, suggests certain criteria of a profession which help us in our present task. Taking first the established professions, the authors make this statement: 'The practitioners, by virtue of prolonged and specialized intellectual training, have acquired a technique which enables them to render a specialized service to the community. This service they perform for a fixed remuneration whether by way of fee or salary. They develop a sense of responsibility for the technique which they manifest in their concern for the competence and honour of the practitioners as a whole—a concern which is sometimes shared with the State. They build up associations, upon which they erect, with or without the co-operation of the State, machinery for imposing tests of competence and enforcing the observance of certain standards of conduct.'[2]

We cannot attempt to consider this whole 'complex of characteristics' in its application to psychiatric social work, but a further statement gives us a starting point: 'It is the existence of specialized intellectual techniques, acquired as the result of prolonged training, which gives rise to professionalism and accounts for its peculiar features.'[3] It is important in any context to know how the word 'technique' is used. Bertha Reynolds, in her *Learning and Teaching in Social Case-work*, defines it for the purposes of her book as: 'The *best way* of doing something—a method which is learned by repeated practice and performed without substantial variation, except as conditions demand the selection of another and probably equally well-learned technique. Techniques are appropriate for activities which lend themselves to standardization and in which originality of method is wasteful rather than desirable.' She adds that 'social work has had relatively few procedures which could be standardized.'[4] It seems clear that the term 'technique' is used by Carr-Saunders and Wilson in a very much wider sense. In one passage the word 'competence' is substituted, a term which certainly covers more than the 'technique' of Bertha Reynolds' definition. Perhaps we may be allowed to avoid controversy by taking the word 'technique' in the present context

[1] Carr-Saunders, A. M., and Wilson, P. A., *The Professions*, Oxford University Press, 1933.

[2] *ibid.*, p. 284.

[3] *ibid.*, pp. 284–5.

[4] Reynolds, Bertha Capen: *Learning and Teaching in the Practice of Social Casework*, Farrar & Rinehart, N.Y., 1942, pp. 51–2.

simply in the sense of that which enables members of a profession to render specialized service to the community, or, in other words, their characteristic form of professional competence.

The question of what constitutes the characteristic competence of psychiatric social work runs through this book. We do not propose to pursue it further here, but rather to consider in relation to this work the statement of Carr-Saunders and Wilson that professional technique is acquired 'by virtue of prolonged and specialized training'. We have suggested earlier that there is nothing incompatible between a sense of vocation and membership of a profession, yet in passing from the first conception to the second we pass to a new range of ideas—those concerned with the disciplined pursuit of knowledge and skill. The conception of training is not implicit in that of vocation, even though any individual who at the present day enters social work with a sense of vocation is likely to be fully aware of the need for it.[1] In the conception of a profession, however, the acquisition of knowledge and skill under regulated conditions is fundamental, and is the profession's justification for tendering its specialized service. Co-operative responsibility for knowledge is the keynote of an article by Dr. John Rickman[2] in which he distinguishes professionalism from quackery. Of the four criteria of a quack he places first the fact that the quack has not submitted himself 'to a course of training regarded as adequate by the teachers in that profession'. He goes on to describe the quack as making 'no consistent endeavour to integrate any discovery he may make in the exercise of the profession to the body of knowledge already existing—to the end that the range of experience of the next generation of students may be improved', adding that these criteria turn on 'willingness to learn in due humility from an older generation' and 'to give, without arrogance, to the next.'

Upon the statements of Carr-Saunders and Wilson and of Rickman we shall base three questions: first, whether the particular service offered to the community by psychiatric social workers can be said to be the outcome of prolonged and specialized training; second, whether they accept responsibility for the

[1] The combination of a strong sense of vocation with a clear conception of the necessity of professional training is illustrated in the life of Florence Nightingale. See Smith, Cecil Woodham: *Florence Nightingale*, Constable, 1950, *passim*, but especially pp. 17 and 483.

[2] Rickman, John, 'Psychology in Medical Education', *British Medical Journal*, September 6, 1947, p. 363, footnote.

increasing of knowledge within their own sphere; third, whether they accept responsibility for making available such knowledge as they possess, vertically to each new generation preparing to enter the work, and horizontally to those already qualified. These questions may all be regarded as matters of professional 'competence', although the last is also concerned with professions as confraternities. The question of 'honour', in the sense of 'standards of conduct', we have reserved for later discussion.

Before considering whether training for psychiatric social work in this country is of a length and character which stamps it as professional, we ought to make clear what we regard as the goal of this training; in doing so we shall be summarizing what is stated or implied in many other parts of this book. We do not think that the service for which the training prepares is that of a technician, although technique will play its part where it is appropriate. We think of it rather as the application within the field of mental hygiene of a certain way of seeing things—of seeing the individual and his environment (personal, social, cultural, material) always as one whole, of which the parts act upon and react to each other. Out of this way of seeing will arise appropriate ways of doing, according to the varied situations which arise. The nature of the service rendered is influenced by the fact that psychiatric social work has developed and is usually practised in close association with psychiatry, but we believe that it has its own sphere of responsibility, which is not contained in that of psychiatry, though it is complementary to it.

It seems obvious that such a service calls for wide and liberal training so that the psychiatric social worker may see what she is doing in perspective, against a background of historical change and social movement, and may escape the insidious error that 'wisdom shall die', or was born, with her own or any other generation. How far psychiatric social work in this country is indeed based upon this type of liberal training is not easy to decide. Compared[1] with the increasingly systematized preparation of the social

[1] It is easy to give a wrong impression when comparing training in U.S.A. and Great Britain, since much that in this country is characteristic of specialized training for psychiatric social work is embodied in America in training for social work as a whole. This statement should be considered in relation to the Hollis Report (Hollis, Ernest V., and Taylor, Alice L.: *Social Work Education in the United States*, Columbia University Press, 1951). This Report contains much which it would have been interesting to relate to our own approach to the same or kindred topics; but this did not prove possible.

worker in U.S.A. British training may appear almost casual. At present the specialized training offered by the three Courses in Great Britain lasts for one year only, and behind that lies great variety. Can the preparation which is obligatory for qualification as a psychiatric social worker be regarded as 'prolonged and specialized training', as these words are used in the first of our quotations? We do not think that it can.

One of the referees of our study, a tutor in a social science department of a university, puts the case, though reluctantly, for greater uniformity. She writes: 'For the more general recognition of the psychiatric social worker as a specialist, it seems desirable that she should hold a degree in a subject in the social science group as well as a social science and mental health certificate so that her qualifications may equate to those of the medical team.' She tends at present, in the writer's experience, to be depreciated by local authorities and the medical profession, as having a training which is non-specific, so that she cannot pull her weight in a clinical team. This point cannot be disregarded. On the other hand it would seem to us most unfortunate if any kind of training came to be adopted not because it was intrinsically the best for psychiatric social workers but because of the extrinsic advantages it might bring in co-operating with workers of other disciplines. Perhaps the matter needs to be approached in a different way.

Might it not be claimed that because of the nature of psychiatric social work the preparation for it should be to some extent non-specific, including not only formal training but a variety of types of social experience? The aim of the period of formal training would then be to help the student to understand and integrate this experience and to prepare her to make continuous use in her practice of all experience which may come to her, outside and inside her professional career. This is open to criticism, but not on the grounds of asking too little. Training for psychiatric social work should not, in our view, be imitative; it must be judged on its suitability for psychiatric social work itself. We must now turn to the way those engaged in it view their own functions and shoulder their corporate responsibilities—and first to the increasing of knowledge, within their own sphere.

A subject had entered the Mental Health Course at an unusually early age, straight from a university. Her psychiatrist referee, thinking of the valuable contribution which this highly intelligent worker was able to make in a research post, which she took up as soon as she had qualified, suggested that if her entry into the Course had been delayed a few years, the fresh mind and the enterprise which she brought to research 'would probably have been subdued into concern with routine case-work.' Following up this suggestion, we noted that none of the five subjects who had passed straight from training to a research post had held a post in social work before admission. On the other hand our study showed that some who have been engaged after qualification for a considerable time in clinical work, and so might have been 'subdued into concern with routine case-work', do in fact turn to research. Opportunity and personality both play their part. For one subject, a period of full-time research came in the midst of a career of an unusually wide range; after two years she returned to the clinical post from which she had been seconded. Two subjects, when interviewed, had recently turned to research as a means of standing back from the personal problems which their posts in clinical work had stirred up. In another instance research seemed to represent intellectual compensation to someone who, to her lasting regret, had missed the opportunity of studying for a university degree.

In contrast to this we found a few traces of a definite repudiation of research, almost a fear of becoming involved in it. One subject, who before applying for the Course had held a post as social field worker in a piece of medical research and had entered the Course with the intention of pursuing some kind of research after she had qualified, described how her feelings had changed during training, so that she was no longer willing to engage in research at the expense of case-work. Three others, in dealing with a list of activities which included research, were emphatic: 'Not interested', 'Don't like it'; 'I *would* be most reluctant to undertake any'. All three were qualified academically above the general level of psychiatric social workers, and one had had experience of scholarly research in another field before she qualified.

The possibility of discovery among practising psychiatric social workers is not, of course, confined to posts wholly or largely concerned with research. Among the subjects of our study there were many who were well aware of the wealth of material for advancing psychiatric-social knowledge which lay all around them, upon which they might have worked if they had had the time. The working conditions of most psychiatric social workers rule out research on a large scale, and in most cases it would need great enthusiasm and persistence to carry out any scheme of research at all. Yet we do not think that the comparatively small number of those attempting to forward discovery is altogether accounted for by external conditions.

Such work is going on to a limited extent. A few psychiatric social workers in clinical posts have been able to undertake a definite piece of research in association with a psychiatrist, taking a responsible share in the work. But in some investigations, loosely termed research, where psychiatric social workers follow up certain groups of patients discharged from mental hospitals (such as those who have undergone one of the new forms of physical therapy), their part seems to have been confined to one or more home visits, with little share in the planning of the inquiry or responsibility for interpreting their own findings. The question of initiative and responsibility in psychiatric-social research is necessarily a difficult one, as the report of a referee on a subject employed in full time research suggests. He describes how during the latter part of her period of research she began to find it rather irksome not to be in charge of the inquiry she was carrying out. She had, however, 'no sociological or research experience to enable her to conduct the inquiry independently. . . . Faults therefore lay partly in her training which had not prepared her for independent conduct of research[1] at a fairly high level, and partly in the choice of her subjects, which were as a rule so largely medical that she did not command the necessary knowledge for analysing the findings.'

To sum up what we have learned from our study, we would suggest that while certain psychiatric social workers are eager for an opportunity, at some period of their career, to devote themselves fully to research, and while others recognize its importance and are aware of the wealth of material for genuinely psychiatric-social research that surrounds them in their posts, it cannot be taken for granted that as a body they feel the increasing of knowledge in their own sphere as a corporate responsibility. A few seemed to show a fear of becoming entangled in it. There were several subjects, however, who expressed an attraction to research provided that it grew naturally out of case-work and could be carried on without detriment to it. This is never in practice an

[1] We do not think that it is customary for professional training courses to do more than enable practitioners to appraise the value of different kinds of evidence in their own field. For training in research methods a longer period would be needed.

easy matter, since there is a danger that both case-work and research may be distorted if not pursued with a single eye. Yet serving the need of individuals and the advancement of knowledge within a profession cannot ultimately be incompatible. This is a subject to which the Association of Psychiatric Social Workers might give further attention. When Rickman writes of a 'consistent endeavour to integrate any discovery he (the practitioner) may make in the exercise of the profession to the body of knowledge already existing,' we may assume that it is of wayside discoveries rather than deliberate research that he is thinking.

We come now to the third question, of whether psychiatric social workers accept responsibility for making available the knowledge they possess to those in training and those already qualified. It is worth reminding ourselves of what happens when a new profession is developing. There is likely to be an increase, at least up to a certain point, in the numbers trained each year. In psychiatric social work this has been reflected in the establishment of two additional training courses and also in the use of additional centres of practical training by the original course. Meanwhile, successive generations qualify and in due course become experienced. Some of these stand out as having an aptitude for making their knowledge and experience available to others. Of these some will play their part in the training of students. In psychiatric social work a few take their place as tutors on the staff of the mental health courses and considerably more are engaged, either throughout the year or during the final months, in the supervision of students in practical work at recognized clinics or hospitals. Thus through the increase in the number of those who have themselves passed through the training, tested its value as a preparation for the work they have actually been called upon to do, and, finally, themselves accepted the responsibility of teaching, there flows back into the training courses an increasing volume of professional experience, through which they are kept in touch with the demands of things as they are.

Our study yielded a small amount of material bearing upon how psychiatric social workers regard student supervision. It is clear that it cannot be taken for granted that this responsibility will be welcomed whole-heartedly by everyone. We noticed that, in the schedule in which subjects were asked to rate their own achievement in various activities, supervision of students tended to be rated low. It was often clear that this reflected a highly responsible attitude towards this duty and a correspondingly high standard in assessing one's own work. This was no matter for surprise; what we were less prepared to find was subjects, admittedly few, who regarded supervision as tiresome, or whose interest depended markedly on the personality and capacity of individual students. On the other hand we found two for whom supervision added greatly to the satisfaction of their posts; obviously they enjoyed the stimulus of having to develop a new kind of professional skill.

It is important to remember that students can make their impact upon a profession before they enter it, above all through the process of self-examination and clarification which they tend to set in motion among those who train them. In psychiatric social work, where students are often people of experience and maturity, it might be expected that this advance influence on practice would be felt to a considerable degree; we found some evidence of this. Indeed the distinction which we have made between vertical communication from the qualified to the not yet qualified, and horizontal among the qualified is somewhat of an abstraction, and certainly does not do justice to the interplay which in fact takes place between those engaged in training and those being trained.

While in a very real sense all those who are qualified are on a professional level, it is obvious that in psychiatric social work there will exist differences of experience and aptitudes. The fact that in this country we have no system of formal supervision beyond the period of student training does not mean that there is not a great deal of passing on of professional knowledge by the more to the less experienced. From the latter, as from the student, will come to the more experienced worker the stimulus to re-think old problems and even a challenge to break up long-established patterns of professional practice. Some of the newly qualified may keep an informal contact with their training through tutor or supervisor; some, in posts where more than one psychiatric social worker is employed, will draw upon the experience of senior colleagues; others again will seek out, in unofficial ways, individuals in their profession with that kind of wisdom through which the less experienced can learn. Moreover, the influence of the professional association now comes directly into play.

All this may be criticized as too fortuitous. It certainly throws much responsibility upon the Association of Psychiatric Social Workers, whose work in stimulating the interchange of knowledge and ideas amongst its members can only be judged when the work of sub-committees and local branches is fully appreciated. Yet it is easy for the need to meet urgent practical tasks and problems to override in this body the discussion of matters of skill, knowledge and principle which are of more lasting concern. When, in 1947, the *British Journal of Psychiatric Social Work* was established, it was hoped by many that it would prove a valuable additional means of communication on these matters. Up to the time of writing (1952) there has been no evidence among psychiatric social workers of a strong desire to write for it. It represents, nevertheless, a step in the breaking down of the British social worker's notorious reluctance to write about what she is doing, and already a number of questions of genuine professional interest have been aired.

iii

We hope that the picture of psychiatric social work which has emerged so far has shown a body of people engaged in work which deserves the name of professional and increasingly called upon to assume professional responsibilities. Up to the present we have confined ourselves to questions relating to professional competence. We would now turn to that aspect of professionalism referred to by Carr-Saunders and Wilson when they write of a profession's 'concern for the . . . honour of the practitioners as a whole', and of the observance of certain standards of professional conduct.

In recent years a desire has shown itself among social workers of various countries to formulate a professional code. In this country a group of social workers in 1950 issued a draft statement of obligations under the headings: to the client, to the community, to the profession.[1] To these general obligations psychiatric social workers would, we believe, be able to subscribe. In what follows we shall be more concerned with particular issues which meet them in challenging forms in the specialized work which they are doing.

If we accept the definition of ethics as conduct considered from the standpoint of value, professional ethics must of course be regarded as subscribing to and governed by moral values of a wider range, which lie beyond the scope of this inquiry. Yet those who,

[1] See 'A Code for Professional Social Work', *Social Work*, October 1950, pp. 490–4. Wider ground was covered at a conference of the Association of Social Workers in 1952 on 'The Social Worker and the Social Conscience'.

as psychiatric social workers, undertake responsibility in connexion with mentally handicapped individuals are inevitably faced with certain problems of value which arise out of their profession and these are at least as complex as those of fact. One of the most important functions of training is to provide the opportunity for clear thinking about such issues. Students of the Mental Health Course may be confronted at an early stage with such questions as the sterilization of mental defectives or criminal responsibility. Moreover in their own case-work they are not unlikely to find themselves, at the first interview, concerned with important questions of right and wrong as well as with problems of knowledge and skill.

It is possible for the psychiatric social worker to be involved simultaneously in many allegiances—to the patient and to the members of his human environment, to the organization in which she works, to the psychiatrist with whom she is directly associated, to the community in a special sense in her capacity as a social worker, and these by no means exhaust the list. We do not want to exaggerate the complexity of her position; nevertheless it is true to say that she is confronted with ethical problems which, akin as they are to those found in medicine and social work respectively, can only be worked out in accordance with that particular amalgam which she represents.

In an earlier chapter we referred to problems of professional conduct encountered in the war years in conditions which were not conducive to clear thinking. Looking back it would seem that the time for clear thinking by the profession as a whole about what may be called professional ethics has been perpetually deferred through a succession of urgent practical demands. This is not necessarily a bad thing, since experience in a number of situations has given the Association and its individual members material to work on which could only have been amassed in the course of years. Perhaps the time has come when the subject can be profitably explored.

In calling for a reconsideration of professional ethics in the medical profession Dr. T. F. Fox, to whose two lectures on 'Professional Freedom'[1] we are greatly indebted in this section, wrote as follows: 'The formulation of rules is really far less important than the cultivation of a professional attitude in the young men and women who will succeed to our heritage. By a professional

[1] Fox, T. F., 'Professional Freedom', Croonian Lectures for 1951, printed in the *Lancet*, July 21st, pp. 115–19, and 28th, pp. 171–5, 1951.

attitude I certainly do not mean loyalty to the profession for its own sake; like the State itself, our profession is not an entity with rights of its own, but merely a means to an end. Still less do I mean that the future doctor should develop a highly specialised outlook on life. . . . If we really intend to preserve professional freedom to any good purpose, the first essential is to produce doctors evidently worthy to have it.'[1] In an earlier paragraph Dr. Fox had already turned upon his own title, suggesting that 'what we seek is not so much professional freedom (which has a selfish ring), as professional responsibility.'[2]

Placing the chief emphasis upon the worker's responsibility to the client, where, among these many allegiances, we should all agree it belongs, we would raise first the question of respecting the client's confidence. The psychiatric social worker attached to hospital or clinic inherits the advantages of the community's assumption that secrets confided to any medical practitioner or medical institution will be respected, and is, of course, herself bound by this tradition. Because, however, her work brings her into more direct touch with the patient's human environment than does the doctor's, and because her duties, especially in work with adults, include the mobilization of the community's resources to meet the patient's needs, she is faced with problems which are different from his and akin to, yet not identical with, those of her fellow social workers.

The fact that the psychiatric social worker, in her characteristic capacity, is dealing with mental illness and disorders of behaviour crucially affects the ethical problems she has to face. It may be true (though experience makes one very cautious in asserting it) that mental illness should be, and in the future will be, regarded with no more fear, shame or social sensitiveness than any other form of illness. That time has certainly not yet come, and this fact, together with the intrinsic nature of the human ills with which she deals and the highly confidential character of the information to which her attachment to clinic or hospital gives her access, demands a degree of discretion which cannot too often be called to mind.

When, as representative of her hospital or clinic, she approaches other social workers or administrative officers in the welfare services whose help she wishes to enlist on the patient's behalf, ques-

[1] *ibid.*, July 28th, pp. 174–5.
[2] *ibid.*, July 21st, p. 119.

tions arise which are rooted in her dual rôle. When the psychiatrist himself deals directly with a social agency, he will sometimes show such reserve that the members of the agency's staff feel that knowledge is being withheld from them which it is important for them to have if they are to help the patient effectively. It is not unnatural that they should feel obstructed and at times resentful. It will often fall to the psychiatric social worker to supplement in personal discussion the hospital's official report. Yet her hands are not free. She can only act as a member of the staff of the hospital and in accordance with its general policy. She is fully bound by the tradition on which the community's faith in medical discretion is based. At the same time, however, as a social worker she is in a position to understand the agency's viewpoint and needs.

This does not mean that she will always be able to dispel the agency's sense of being shut out by the hospital from knowledge which it ought to have or the suspicion which sometimes arises that the psychiatric social worker herself is being possessive about a case, as indeed she may sometimes be. Yet a sincere admission of the difficulties inherent in this form of co-operation can do much, above all perhaps the recognition that the agency worker, no less than herself, can only help a client within a sound professional relationship. The more widely the importance of the relationship between social worker and client comes to be understood, the more effectively should social workers of different services be able to work together in such a situation, yet not necessarily easily. Special justification is needed for infringing the client's right to privacy and this must never be sacrificed to facilitate relations between social workers. Such situations, honestly faced, will rarely be altogether free from strain.

When the passing on of certain information not of a strictly medical kind seems essential if the agency is to play its part, then it is often possible for the psychiatric social worker to get the patient's permission to do this or to get him to understand the importance of doing it himself. This is indeed the most common solution of such problems, when the patient is reasonably capable of directing his own affairs. But the psychiatric social worker, with her strong conviction of the right of every individual to self-direction, has committed herself to a profession which involves her in the service of many who, at least temporarily, are unable to exercise that right. Some of her more difficult problems of professional ethics are bound up with this. We have described a way of working which we referred to as the psychiatric social worker's chosen method. It sometimes happens, especially in work with adults, that she is called upon to undertake duties which involve methods very remote from it. We have referred to her dismay when it was first suggested that she should act as duly authorized officer under the Lunacy and Mental Treatment Acts. A comparable situation, though perhaps less openly challenging, faces the psychiatric social worker in a mental observation ward, when a patient is brought in who is unable to give any account of himself and about whom information is required for the assessment of both his psychiatric and social needs. For the time being she may have to play something of a detective's part. If she is satisfied that such work is necessary, and that it is appropriate that she should undertake it, then it seems to us important that she should assume those duties frankly and not apologetically. Only then is she likely to expend upon them her full knowledge and skill, and bring them fully within the sphere of her professional ethics.

It is not as easy as one would like to believe to ensure that one's decision whether or not to intervene professionally, and in what way, rests entirely upon the needs of the patient and his human environment and not upon one's own need to dominate, either by depriving the patient of responsibility which he is capable of assuming, or (a more subtle form of the same need) by forcing upon him, on theoretical grounds, responsibility for which he is unfit. It is possible for repudiation of responsibility on the worker's part in certain circumstances to result in less rather than greater freedom for the patient. A seriously depressed patient left with the burden of some personal decision may present a mere caricature of a free person. This is an extreme case, yet certain risks, known and unknown, are involved wherever human liberty is at stake. There is indeed no situation in which purely theoretical considerations, indiscriminately applied, are less in place than where a worker is trying to weigh the ability of a client at a particular point of time to shoulder responsibility for directing his own life.

The question of responsibility has many facets. A psychiatric social worker remarked to one of us that we belonged to a profession in which we must always be prepared to get into trouble. There is some truth in this, yet we wonder whether we always make due allowance for the possibility of 'trouble' which is the psychiatrist's daily companion. This sometimes accounts for a psychiatric social worker's irritation at what she regards as the psychiatrist's over-cautious attitude, which she sees as obstructing her own work in a case. It seems to us important that she should try to understand as fully as possible the psychiatrist's position in this regard. Entering the field of psychiatry as a lay worker, while she can add to the psychiatrist's 'trouble' she cannot share his ultimate responsibility, in so far as this depends upon his being a doctor. We do not think that any psychiatric social worker would question the psychiatrist's assumption of this responsibility for patients suffering from mental illness, and in this we are not only thinking of the functions vested in him by law as a 'duly qualified medical practitioner'. The question of medical direction of child guidance clinics is a matter of discussion into which we ourselves do not feel called upon to enter. We have referred to a scheme put forward by a psychiatrist for the working of a clinic team, in which the responsibility for the care and treatment of patients would be vested in the team, the psychiatrist 'permitting to his colleagues full therapeutic autonomy, whilst being prepared at any moment to assume the full responsibility for the conduct of any case'. The social worker should not underestimate what this entails for the psychiatrist.

T. F. Fox in the lectures already quoted makes the doctor's responsibility for the individual patient the touchstone of his professional character. If we accept this, does it imply that we give up all claim to professional standing because the ultimate responsibility for the management of a case lies elsewhere? If not, what is the nature and extent of the responsibility proper to us as psychiatric social workers? In an earlier chapter we represented a group of psychiatric social workers strongly repudiating the honourable analogy of a pathologist who has been brought into a case by the psychiatrist in charge. Apt as such an analogy might appear at first sight, we regard its rejection as both understandable and healthy, chiefly perhaps because it implies a fragmentation which the psychiatric social worker feels to be quite alien to the kind of service she is best fitted to offer. With her special concern for the 'body social' within which the patient is, as it were, embedded, the psychiatric social worker cannot do her best work when a case is referred to her by a psychiatrist for a narrowly limited piece of social service and without freedom to use her judgment about the whole of the social aspect of a patient's needs and of the implications of any social action taken.

The point at which the worker herself is perhaps most deeply aware of her own inescapable responsibility is in the relationship which, whatever may be the task to be undertaken between them, she aims to establish with some individual forming part of the texture of a case, in child guidance usually with the mother of the child patient, in work with adults with either patient or relative. That the psychiatrist should understand and respect this is an important condition of her work. In the case of an adult patient still under psychiatric treatment it is obviously desirable that the situation of the patient's dual relation, to psychiatrist on the one side and to the social worker on the other, should be clearly understood between the two, and that this understanding should be shared to some degree by the patient. In child guidance it is safe to assume that the social worker's professional relation with the parent of the child patient is normally accepted by the team as a whole.

If we claim that the relations which we establish with clients as a basis of our work should be respected, as a serious part of our professional service, it is for us to consider the quality of these relations. Naturally, we do not suggest that our obligations differ essentially from those encumbent upon any professional person working with individuals. It is rather that in psychiatric social work, where technical and other practical services to the individual are apt to be at a minimum, the relationship itself is left in relief, and so calls specially for scrutiny. No one would question the obligation of any professional person to ensure that their relationship with the person served was immune from material self-interest on the side of the former. The probation officer in an unnamed county who was found by one of us to be using his visits to further his own interests as an estate agent, and the public servant who is not able to distinguish personal from professional relationships when his duties involve social occasions, are condemned without question. Even salaries for social work were regarded as suspect by our forbears. It is far less easy, but no less important, to see that the client is protected from the personal vested interests of the case-worker of a subtler kind.

Because both client and worker may be to a great extent unaware of what is going on, to press 'invisible wares' upon a client in a professional relationship can do more damage than traffic in real estate. We have considered in an earlier chapter the importance to the client of the worker's having herself some consistent attitude to life and the equal importance of her not imposing upon him her own convictions. To steer a course between the two, with the needs of the client, as they gradually reveal themselves in the process of the developing relationship, as the undeviatingly pursued goal may come easily to some workers. To others this may present an insoluble problem, since their own convictions include the conviction that they know the client's needs and can supply them. We have already suggested that this attitude is hardly compatible with the assumptions upon which psychiatric social work is based, and we believe that it is the business of selection to forestall the difficulties which are likely to arise if people such as we have described are admitted to train for it.

Yet we doubt whether there is any one of us who has never allowed an ulterior motive to enter a professional relationship. To some of us the problem presents itself as the difficulty of preserving, in those free conditions of work which most of us particularly value, a professional relationship of which the nature is understood by the client. A relationship which the client misinterprets as being a personal one, so that it has to be brought back to a professional level and its real nature underlined, may cause not only distress which should have been avoided, but also actual harm, especially to a client in whom there has begun to develop a pattern of life in which he sees himself as recurrently 'let down'. Such misunderstandings always challenge the worker to consider whether an ulterior motive may not have crept into her work, perhaps of the nature of a wish to be appreciated as a person in whom one can confide or as one who does not really subscribe to the tiresome restrictions of the organization which she represents. The offering of gifts by client to worker will sometimes be an indication of how little the client has understood the nature of the professional relationship. It is the business of the worker to ensure that it is implicitly understood, though not necessarily to force it upon the client as an intellectual proposition. This might be more damaging in certain circumstances than the worker's acceptance of a gift. The client in some cases may have a compelling need to turn a professional into a personal relationship; most psychiatric social workers could illustrate this from their dealings with hysterical patients. To understand the nature of this need and to help the client to understand it and to use the forces behind it belong to the worker's professional competence. To avoid becoming entangled in any of the subtle flattery which such a situation contains for the worker herself is a matter of professional ethics. Those who have been professionally trained are unlikely to fall a prey to the cruder forms of temptation to unprofessional attitudes and conduct, but in real situations these appear in insidious forms and can easily pass undetected.

A large range of unprofessional motives may enter into the taking of a social history. When, as often happens, such a history is called for in the first place in order to help the psychiatrist in diagnosis, the situation is much more complicated than when, in a social agency, a worker builds up a social history primarily as a basis for her own future work or for the work of someone of the same discipline as herself. With the psychiatric social worker this purpose is always present; at the same time the psychiatrist's need for her contribution to diagnosis imposes upon her certain conditions, such as those of speed and in some cases of a more direct pursuit of information than she would have used were she not working in this relation with psychiatry. These are problems which are comparatively well defined and on which it should be possible to reach some kind of agreement between psychiatrist and psychiatric social worker. Others are more subtle. However good the relation between psychiatrist and social worker may be, the fact that she belongs to a discipline which has not yet altogether moved out of the stage in which it has to demonstrate its value makes her subject to a temptation to produce a 'good' report in the eyes of the psychiatrist. In one sense, of course, this is what every psychiatric social worker would try to do and such an ambition produces useful results. But if the psychiatric social worker is to be a professional worker, it is essential that her sense of responsibility for the effect of the history taking upon those from whom she obtains it should take precedence over any wish for the approbation of the psychiatrist or any other member of the team in which she works.

It is easy to deceive oneself, just because many of the motives, which are impermissible if allowed to usurp the first place, are useful as auxiliaries. It is good for a case-worker to be competent, and even to enjoy her competence, but if case-work comes to be valued as a means of exercising it, there is always a danger of its becoming dehumanized. Again case-work may be more satisfactory to both client and worker if each has a liking for the other. A mature professional worker, who finds that she shares with a client a common interest, may use this as a means of easing the first contact, and, in its proper place, throughout the whole development of a case, provided that her work is firmly based upon a disinterested concern for the client's welfare. A relationship based upon liking or a common interest will hardly bear the strain of the serious personal problems which will have to be worked out within it, or the hostility of client to worker which may need to be uncovered as the case develops.

It would not be difficult to extend this list of unprofessional elements which are always ready to insinuate themselves into psychiatric social work. For all of us temptation probably lies chiefly in the region of the relation between worker and client, and the importance which we attach to this makes it especially encumbent upon us to examine ourselves in this respect. There is a sense in which relations are all important; within a sound relationship mistakes can be retrieved and damage made good. This is recognized in the bringing up of children. Yet this is dangerous doctrine unless it is recognized as involving something which is immensely difficult to achieve. Aristotle's 'Between friends there is no need of justice' and St. Augustine's 'Love, and do as thou wilt', which in a perfect world would make all professional codes unnecessary, imply a quality of friendship and of love which we cannot take for granted in professional relations. For this reason most of us, who do not find it easy to maintain consistently the standards of decent professional people, are glad to be supported by professional 'obligations' against which we can measure ourselves from time to time. To keep a constant and conscious watch in the actual course of one's case-work against any tendency to subtle exploitation could easily kill spontaneity. Most of us know ourselves well enough to be aware at what points we are most liable to fall short of our professional standards. It is wiser to accept in humility the fact that we are unlikely to pass through our career with our professional motives unmixed.

It seems a fair summary of the present situation to say that psychiatric social workers, individually and as a body, are seeking to ensure conditions of work in which they may assume greater responsibility for their own functions, and to say further that, when they do this, they are giving evidence of increasing professional maturity, even when there may be differences of opinion about the form the responsibility should take. The Mackintosh Report gives assurance that their growing acceptance of professional responsibility corresponds to an external demand that they should assume it. In the meantime there is no lack of wide questions with ethical implications on which the corporate judgment of psychiatric social workers can exercise itself. One of the psychiatrist referees already quoted suggests in his report that the profession has a responsibility 'for the total environment of the sick (i.e., mentally sick) at whatever level or by whatever means it may require modification'. Before a profession is ready to consider its duties in this comprehensive way it must have reached a certain stage of development. Our professional training, as we have shown, was certainly not established on the basis of any single defined conception such as this. But the problem presented by this referee has much in common with those which face psychiatric social workers in the Mackintosh Report and cannot be evaded. The 'extremely erratic distribution' of such psychiatric social workers as there are, referred to in paragraph 63 of the Report, is a problem about which the Association might feel some kind of corporate responsibility. It exists, of course, in the medical profession also. The principle involved is summed up by Fox in a sentence which is full of suggestion for our own profession. After reiterating that doctors, for the public good, must remain the servants of their patients and personally responsible for their work, he admits that 'In their individualism, so largely beneficial, doctors have often been myopic in their outlook—and too little interested in the needs of those people with whom they are not personally confronted. Granted that our task is to serve human beings and not policies . . . . we still have a duty to see that our knowledge is used as widely and as wisely as the times permit'.[1]

It is to be noted that the author of the lectures on 'Professional Freedom' is not greatly concerned about whether those who claim professional status have proved their claim. We do not claim to have proved our own. The demand for professional or semi-professional status ought, he thinks, to be satisfied since, in 'a world of obscure meaning in which, without faith, it is hard even to tell right from wrong . . . the professions . . . are channels for an increasing flow of altruistic effort. . . . For professionalism, with all its faults, has proved to be one of the major civilising influences of our times.'[2]

The conception of a profession as a 'channel', which prevents something valuable from seeping away, is significant. A channel is open at both ends. It does not serve its purpose if it is shut in upon itself. It is not inconceivable that the contours of the social field

[1] *ibid.*, July 28th, p. 175.
[2] *ibid.*, July 21st, p. 115.

may change in such a way that the channel of psychiatric social work will no longer be necessary, at least in anything like its present form. It is possible that in more propitious circumstances many of the values canalized could, without loss, be allowed to flow more widely over the land. To accept the possibility of a metamorphosis into something at present unpredictable need not discourage the profession from a persistent attempt to discover its true nature and to develop it to the full. Every profession which aims at helping to alleviate human suffering or to meet human needs works towards its own extinction. Psychiatric social work, sharing this distant aim, must also, perhaps, accept the possibility of transformation at a less Utopian range. A marked rise in the level of training in general social work, especially in case-work, might affect the future of psychiatric social work in a fundamental way, though it would not, we believe, make it unnecessary as a specialized service. Such a speculative future is stimulating and enlarging to the mind. In the meantime we may be well content to play a part with other professional and semi-professional bodies in this civilizing influence, and grateful to find the respectability of altruism taken so simply for granted.

CHAPTER XII

CONCLUSION

THIS book is concerned with a single branch of social work. Our study of it, however, has led us to certain considerations which may have wider significance. We shall try to draw them together in this chapter and leave it to our readers to judge.

While this book has been in the making much thought has been given to training for social work as a whole, and in particular to the trend towards specialization of which psychiatric social work is only one example. We share the view expressed in the Mackintosh and Younghusband reports that the time has come to consider whether the present effort to meet the needs of different services by particular courses of training is well spent. Much might be gained from a common vocational training based upon degree or diploma courses in social science. The whole teaching of the study and treatment of human relations needs to be thought out again in the light of advancing knowledge and the changes in social services. We have much to learn from the United States and from Canada, where psychiatric social workers are no longer regarded as a group exercising a special skill, and where those who set out to offer services to families, to dependent children, to sick people or to delinquents share to a large extent the same professional study and discipline. One thing at least seems clear, that however desirable it may be for these groups of social workers to explore human problems in common, each group would also need to gain experience and exact knowledge bearing upon its own branch of service; otherwise what was gained from learning together might be offset by too much generality. In our view this double need would not be satisfactorily met merely by adding the special to the general study, but only by a judicious combination of the two kinds of learning.

Our own experience as well as our special study have convinced us that professional training for social work, however specialized, should continue to be regarded as a form of liberal education and not as the learning of techniques. Disciplined thought is essential to that philosophic outlook without which social work is liable to develop into a mere application of devices for meeting immediate social problems. Personal attitudes cannot be divorced from the mastery of facts and the development of discriminating judgment. If this is true of general education it is still more true in preparing for a vocation concerned with human beings, in which knowledge cannot be safely used except by those who are on the way to mastering the vagaries of individual thought and feeling. This is not to suggest that education should be confused with therapy. It is the job of the educator to help the student to use both emotion and reason in the process of learning; if personal problems interfere with this then they should be treated elsewhere.

We have discussed the variety to be found in the equipment of those who entered the Mental Health Course as we knew it. Such variety undoubtedly sets special problems for those engaged in training. Yet our study convinced us that a wide range of personal qualities and experiences can be used with success in this work. Loss of the pliability and resilence characteristic of the young may be compensated for by the greater wealth of wisdom of those who have stood the test of responsibility in other kinds of work. Those who select must therefore beware of their tendency to look for certain types of persons rather than for qualities found in very varying combination. Standards there must be, but perhaps the essential skill of those who select for this kind of work lies in the power to recognize the individual's capacity for growth through experience of every sort. Such skill must include ability to assess the meaning of personal difficulties through which the candidate for training has passed, and for this the advice of a psychiatrist may be needed. Our study does not suggest that personal disturbance is necessarily to be regarded as indicating risks which should never be taken.

The acceptance of variety as desirable means that those responsible for training must be prepared to accept the individual's natural tempo of personal growth and learning. A balance must be found between the essential discipline of a standard of achievement required for any profession and the individual's own peculiar ways of reaching out towards this standard. This implies in the planning of such a course a generous conception of the demands it will make on the training staff, in the time to be devoted directly to individual students, to the unhurried consideration of how to make the training most profitable for each and to frequent consultation between tutors and supervisors. The importance of this personal learning is borne out at every point in our study. It calls for far more thought than has so far been given to it, and there is great need for further opportunity for education of the educators.

We have described a period of professional practice in which psychiatric social workers entering employment have been called upon to fulfil a wide variety of functions and in which there have been many different conceptions of their responsibilities. While this has led to some unrest and uneasiness we see it as a natural characteristic of a new development and perhaps a healthy one. This variety depends in part upon the difference of conditions found, for example, in the child-guidance and mental hospital services. Yet our study brought home to us in how many different ways, within such externally imposed conditions, a job might be carried out. The qualities and experience of the particular psychiatric social worker, her conception of the work she had been trained to do, the interplay between herself and other workers brought into professional association within the service concerned, all these have a bearing upon achievement. It is not irrelevant to point out here that in every profession members are impelled to decide to what extent it is right for them to shape their service according to the quality demanded and paid for by the community and to what extent they must abide by their own developing understanding of its purpose. It is a no less inescapable fact that if the profession is to survive its goods must have a reasonable sale price.

We have discussed what may be termed two kinds of social conscience in psychiatric social work; the one is expressed in concentration upon intensive work on highly selected cases, the other in the acceptance of an obligation towards all those who, directly or indirectly, are in need of what this service has to offer. We believe that the existence within the profession of these two groups is beneficial, provided that the contribution made by each is mutually understood and respected.

Our study provided many illustrations of how deeply the attitude of a psychiatrist to a psychiatric social worker with whom he is associated may influence the character of the work which the social worker is able to carry out. We use the title 'Working in Partnership' for the chapter in which these matters are discussed in order to emphasize the need for these two to work together as professional colleagues. Allowing for the fact that equally good results may be achieved through forms of association which are in appearance very different, we have the impression that not a few psychiatric social workers, especially those working with adult patients, feel discouraged in trying to practise what they believe themselves fitted to undertake by finding themselves in a position nearer to that of an auxiliary[1] than of a professional colleague.

It occurred to us that more thought might be given by psychiatric social workers not only to their own position (which can never be a simple one in view of the dual nature of their training and interest) but also to the characteristic problems and responsibilities of psychiatrists in their medical capacity, by which their own work in association with psychiatry must be to some extent conditioned. Perhaps they might also give more thought to the kind of freedom which they in fact possess and the kind which they would like to have. Thus their comparatively 'extraneous' position in a mental hospital carries both advantages and disadvantages and cannot be understood apart from the fact that, among all those in the hospital service, psychiatric social workers stand in a unique relation to the community outside it, where indeed their professional roots are to be sought. We have considered in various connexions the dual nature of the work which is the subject of our book. This may be a source of considerable conflict in the minds of those who practise it, tempting them to retreat in one or other direction from that point of convergence of psychiatric and social where, in our view, their true strength will always lie.

We have given special attention to criticisms of psychiatric social workers' shortcomings, especially in their relations with those they work with in the field of social service, not only because they themselves feel a special responsibility in human relationships but because others expect much from them in this sphere and are concerned when they fail to live up to these expectations. We suggest how this situation may have arisen and certain means by which, without repudiating their special obligations, psychiatric social workers may come to be regarded in a more realistic way.

Our special study impressed upon us how individual a matter a professional career is, and how the need to allow for a natural tempo of growth by no means ceases with formal training. In the

[1] While we were considering professional relations from the standpoint of this study, there appeared the Cope Report, making the notion of a medical auxiliary an important practical issue. Ministry of Health: *Reports of the Committees on Medical Auxiliaries*, H.M. Stationery Office, 1951.

chapter called 'The Shaping of Careers' we try to show what a wide sweep of experience is often necessary before a person's real quality can be assessed. To admit this is to recognize the importance of being allowed to make one's own vocational mistakes, and precludes any naïve acceptance of vocational guidance as an unmixed blessing, whatever improvements in its techniques the future may hold. This would seem to include the individual's right to experiment in types of work and not only in particular jobs. We have never been able to forget, however, even while we were impressed in many individual cases with the ultimate value of apparently unfortunate experiences, the cost of experimentation in a profession where the material is individual human beings. We have to admit that we have no means of assessing the cost to clients, or to the profession as a whole, of an individual worker's finding herself professionally at her own time and in her own way.

In the careers which we studied there were not a few examples of subjects who qualified and later passed outside the mental health service in its usually accepted sense. Without denying the seriousness of this in a period of severe shortage of qualified workers in this field, we have hesitated to regard this as 'wastage'. While recognizing the value of continuity (within professions, within jobs and in relations between workers and individual clients), we still welcome conditions which allow for mobility, both within psychiatric social work itself and within the wider field of social services to which it belongs.

This book has frequently laid stress upon the value of variety, of flexibility, of allowing things to happen and of being available rather than intervening. This might suggest a form of *laissez-faire* to which we should not in fact wish to subscribe, if we failed to point out that we have also stressed the importance of standards and of imposed conditions in all three phases—selection, training and professional practice. We have also, at least by implication, upheld the importance of planning, especially that which is founded upon such information as we believe to be accumulating amongst us without as yet being turned to account.

In the last chapter we considered the claims of psychiatric social work to be regarded as a profession. We realize that professionalism implies the recognition of boundaries. It seems to us, however, that those engaged in this work are in a particularly good position for remaining aware of the temporary nature of all boundaries which isolate human beings, and that it is important for them to preserve this awareness. A client will thus be seen as accepting her position in relation to a worker for a certain purpose and as long as a certain situation lasts. Again, a candidate for training in psychiatric social work will be seen as someone who may become a student and later a qualified practitioner and so, it may be, herself take part in selection and training for her profession. To do her job well the psychiatric social worker must have, we believe, a deep sense of belonging to the medium in which she works, must keep herself aware of being a potential client or patient and know that she shares with the man in the street much of his ignorance of others' expert knowledge. She must, moreover, be able to turn these things to good account in terms of an understanding of how people feel and think and of what her own behaviour may mean to them.

This positive acceptance of a lay element in the essential character of our work is one side of the picture as we see it. The other is—to adjust Bacon's proud words to the modest scale of our own profession—the need to 'take all knowledge to be our province'. This is clearly not a matter to be dealt with in a year of formal specialized training or indeed in any such training however prolonged. The question of how to consolidate it in ways appropriate to the various needs of those who have passed through it is one which calls for still further consideration and experimentation. It is obviously a complicated one, since it is not only a question of developing further skill in case-work but of keeping psychiatric social workers' abreast of such developments as concern them in the two fields of their dual interests, and these fields may be expected to widen as time goes on.

Sir Richard Livingstone in *The Future of Education*[1] makes a memorable plea for education extending throughout a lifetime. All his arguments can be applied to the importance in work such as our own of a conception of training which is never completed. The detailed problems of how the formal training is to be consolidated can, we believe, be solved if a general belief exists among psychiatric social workers that, in starting to train for their profession, they embark upon a process in which professional and personal experience and its communication and the pursuit of knowledge are in constant interplay and that to this process, within the career of any individual, no bounds can be set.

[1] Livingstone, Richard: *The Future in Education*, Cambridge University Press, 1941.

APPENDIX 1

OCCUPATIONS OF MEMBERS OF THE ASSOCIATION OF PSYCHIATRIC SOCIAL WORKERS LIVING IN THE UNITED KINGDOM, ACCORDING TO THE LIST PUBLISHED BY THE ASSOCIATION IN JANUARY 1951, SUPPLEMENTED BY THE LIST OF APRIL 1952.

This list includes men. Between 83 and 84% of qualified workers are members of the Association.

Type of Work	Description	Number 467	Per cent
MENTAL HEALTH SERVICES		**308**	**65.9**
Child Guidance Clinics	*Includes separate clinics and centres, and out-patient hospital departments for children.*	127	
Mental Hospitals and Psychiatric Centres for Adults	*Includes three institutions for mental defectives.*	107	
Mental Observation Wards		8	
General Hospitals; Psychiatric Out-Patient Clinics for Adults		38	
University Medical Schools: Psychiatric Departments	*Clinical work combined with teaching of staff other than psychiatric social workers.*	4	
Community Care of Mental Patients	*Not attached to clinic. Only four work solely with mental defectives.*	21	
Other Posts	*e.g., vocational guidance, Board of Control inspectorship.*	4	

APPENDIX 1—*continued*

Type of Work	Description	Number 467	Per cent
OTHER TYPES OF SOCIAL SERVICE		**33**	**7.1**
Delinquents	*e.g., prison, probation, approved schools.*	9	
Child Care	*e.g., Home Office inspectorships, childrens' officers, staff of voluntary organizations and childrens' homes.*	18	
Other Posts	*e.g., hospital almoners, family case workers.*	6	
TRAINING STUDENTS		**19**	**4.1**
Psychiatric Social Workers Courses		7	
Other University Courses for Social Workers	*Includes one director of a social science department and four responsible for Child Care Courses.*	8	
Other Training	*e.g., family welfare and staff of Childrens' Homes.*	4	
RESEARCH		**13**	**2.8**
EMPLOYMENT FOR WHICH QUALIFICATION NOT RELEVANT	*Includes posts (e.g., teaching) for which some have regarded the training as useful*	**6**	**1.3**
NO EMPLOYMENT LISTED	*Large proportion married. A number are caring for young children, often after period of employment.*	**88**	**18.8**

APPENDIX 2

LIST OF MOTIVES FOR APPLICATION FOR TRAINING USED IN THE SPECIAL STUDY

Each subject was asked to mark those statements which applied to herself, and to underline those of particular importance in her case.

1	I wanted to have a break from my occupation.	
2	I wanted to have a year at the University.	
3	I wanted to have a year for study.	
4	I wanted to earn a higher salary.	
5	I wanted to improve my professional status.	
6	I wanted to gain a recognized qualification for a job I was already doing, or a job which had been promised me.	
7	I wanted to gain more understanding of the problems I was already meeting in my work.	
8	I wanted to qualify myself to play a part in future developments in the field of mental health.	
9	I wanted to qualify myself for psychiatric social work.	
10	I wanted to help individuals undergoing mental suffering.	
11	I happened to hear about the Mental Health Course.	
12	I wanted to know more about the workings of my own mind.	
13	I wanted to work closely with the medical profession.	
14	I hoped that the Mental Health Course would help me to understand my own psychological difficulties.	
15	Others thought me suitable for psychiatric social work.	
16	I believed I had some natural ability for understanding and helping people.	

INDEX